Applied Longitudinal Data Analysis for Epidemiology

A Practical Guide

In this book the most important techniques available for longitudinal data analysis are discussed. This discussion includes simple techniques such as the paired *t*-test and summary statistics, and also more sophisticated techniques such as generalized estimating equations and random coefficient analysis. A distinction is made between longitudinal analysis with continuous, dichotomous, and categorical outcome variables. The emphasis of the discussion lies in the interpretation of the different techniques and the comparison of the results of different techniques. Furthermore, special chapters deal with the analysis of two measurements, experimental studies and the problem of missing data in longitudinal studies. Finally, an extensive overview of (and a comparison between) different software packages is provided. This practical guide is suitable for non-statisticians and researchers working with longitudinal data from epidemiological and clinical studies.

Dr Jos W. R. Twisk is senior researcher and lecturer in the Department of Clinical Epidemiology and Biostatistics and the Institute for Research in Extramural Medicine, Vrije Universiteit, Medical Centre, Amsterdam

Applied Longitudinal Data Analysis for Epidemiology

A Practical Guide

Jos W. R. Twisk

Vrije Universiteit Medical Centre, Amsterdam

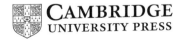

CAMBRIDGE
UNIVERSITY PRESS

PUBLISHED BY THE PRESS SYNDICATE OF THE UNIVERSITY OF CAMBRIDGE
The Pitt Building, Trumpington Street, Cambridge, United Kingdom

CAMBRIDGE UNIVERSITY PRESS
The Edinburgh Building, Cambridge CB2 2RU, UK
40 West 20th Street, New York, NY 10011-4211, USA
477 Williamstown Road, Port Melbourne, VIC 3207, Australia
Ruiz de Alarcón 13, 28014 Madrid, Spain
Dock House, The Waterfront, Cape Town 8001, South Africa

http://www.cambridge.org

First published 2003

Printed in the United Kingdom at the University Press, Cambridge

Typefaces Minion 11/14.5 pt and Formata   *System* LATEX 2$_\varepsilon$ [TB]

A catalogue record for this book is available from the British Library

Library of Congress Cataloguing in Publication data

Twisk, Jos W R, 1962–
Applied longitudinal data analysis for epidemiology : a practical guide / Jos WR Twisk.
   p.   cm.
Includes bibliographical references and index.
ISBN 0-521-81976-8 (hbk). – ISBN 0-521-52580-2 (pbk.)
1. Epidemiology – Research – Statistical methods.   2. Epidemiology – Longitudinal studies.
3. Epidemiology – Statistical methods.   I. Title.
RA652.2.M3 T95   2002
614.4′07′27 – dc21   2002023437

ISBN 0 521 81976 8 hardback
ISBN 0 521 52580 2 paperback

The world is turning, I hope it don't turn away   NEIL YOUNG

To Marjon and Mike

Contents

Preface

The two most important advantages of this book are (1) the fact that it has been written by an epidemiologist, and (2) the word 'applied', which implies that the emphasis of this book lies more on the application of statistical techniques for longitudinal data analysis and not so much on the mathematical background. In most other books on the topic of longitudinal data analysis, the mathematical background is the major issue, which may not be surprising since (nearly) all the books on this topic have been written by statisticians. Although statisticians fully understand the difficult mathematical material underlying longitudinal data analysis, they often have difficulty in explaining this complex material in a way that is understandable for the researchers who have to use the technique or interpret the results. In fact, an epidemiologist is not primarily interested in the basic (difficult) mathematical background of the statistical methods, but in finding the answer to a specific research question; the epidemiologist wants to know how to apply a statistical technique and how to interpret the results. Owing to their different basic interests and different level of thinking, communication problems between statisticians and epidemiologists are quite common. This, in addition to the growing interest in longitudinal studies, initiated the writing of this book: a book on longitudinal data analysis, which is especially suitable for the 'non-statistical' researcher (e.g. epidemiologist). The aim of this book is to provide a practical guide on how to handle epidemiological data from longitudinal studies. The purpose of this book is to build a bridge over the communication gap that exists between statisticians and epidemiologists when addressing the complicated topic of longitudinal data analysis.

Jos Twisk

Amsterdam, January 2002

Acknowledgements

I am very grateful to all my colleagues and students who came to me with (mostly) practical questions on longitudinal data analysis. This book is based on all those questions. Furthermore, I would like to thank Dick Bezemer, Maarten Boers, Bernard Uitdehaag and Wieke de Vente who critically read preliminary drafts of some chapters and provided very helpful comments, and Faith Maddever who corrected the English language.

generalized linear model - charact. by 3 elements: systematic component, link, & random component

    systematic component - same as regular linear model,

    link fcn - describes how expected value of y related to linear predictor

MCAR - missing data process does not depend on the response in any fashion

MAR - missing data " " " " " " unobserved response in any fashion but may depend on previously observed responses

    -only problem for GEE models

MNAR - missing data process does depend on unobserved response

    * a problem for all modeling options

Contin. outcome — multivariate method ok if subjects observed at same fixed time pts & have no missing data, otherwise - use linear mixed model

1

Introduction

1.1 Introduction

Longitudinal studies are defined as studies in which the outcome variable is repeatedly measured; i.e. the outcome variable is measured in the same individual on several different occasions. In longitudinal studies the observations of one individual over time are not independent of each other, and therefore it is necessary to apply special statistical techniques, which take into account the fact that the repeated observations of each individual are correlated. The definition of longitudinal studies (used in this book) implicates that statistical techniques like survival analyses are beyond the scope of this book. Those techniques basically are not longitudinal data analysing techniques because (in general) the outcome variable is an irreversible endpoint and therefore strictly speaking is only measured at one occasion. After the occurrence of an event no more observations are carried out on that particular subject.

Why are longitudinal studies so popular these days? One of the reasons for this popularity is that there is a general belief that with longitudinal studies the problem of causality can be solved. This is, however, a typical misunderstanding and is only partly true. Table 1.1 shows the most important criteria for causality, which can be found in every epidemiological textbook (e.g. Rothman and Greenland, 1998). Only one of them is specific for a longitudinal study: the rule of temporality. There has to be a time-lag between outcome variable Y (effect) and predictor variable X (cause); in time the cause has to precede the effect. The question of whether or not causality exists can only be (partly) answered in specific longitudinal studies (i.e. experimental studies) and certainly not in all longitudinal studies (see Chapter 2). What then is the advantage of performing a longitudinal study? A longitudinal study is expensive, time consuming, and difficult to

Table 1.1. Criteria for causality

Strength of the relationship
Consistency in different populations and under different circumstances
Specificity (cause leads to a single effect)
Temporality (cause precedes effect in time)
Biological gradient (dose–response relationship)
Biological plausibility
Experimental evidence

analyse. If there are no advantages over cross-sectional studies why bother? The main advantage of a longitudinal study compared to a cross-sectional study is that the **individual development** of a certain outcome variable over time can be studied. In addition to this, the **individual development** of a certain outcome variable can be related to the **individual development** of other variables.

1.2 General approach

The general approach to explain the statistical techniques covered in this book will be 'the research question as basis for analysis'. Although it may seem quite obvious, it is important to realize that a statistical analysis has to be carried out in order to obtain an answer to a particular research question. The starting point of each chapter in this book will be a research question, and throughout the book many research questions will be addressed. The book is further divided into chapters regarding the characteristics of the outcome variable. Each chapter contains extensive examples, accompanied by computer output, in which special attention will be paid to interpretation of the results of the statistical analyses.

1.3 Prior knowledge

Although an attempt has been made to keep the complicated statistical techniques as understandable as possible, and although the basis of the explanations will be the underlying epidemiological research question, it will be assumed that the reader has some prior knowledge about (simple) cross-sectional statistical techniques such as linear regression analysis, logistic regression analysis, and analysis of variance.

1.4 Example

In general, the examples used throughout this book will use the same longitudinal dataset. This dataset consists of an outcome variable (Y) that is continuous and is measured six times. Furthermore there are four predictor variables, which differ in distribution (continuous or dichotomous) and in whether they are time dependent or time independent. X_1 is a continuous time-independent predictor variable, X_2 is a continuous time-dependent predictor variable. X_3 is a dichotomous time-dependent predictor variable and X_4 is a dichotomous time-independent predictor variable. All time-dependent predictor variables are measured at the same six occasions as the outcome variable Y.

In some examples a distinction will be made between the example dataset with equally spaced time intervals and a dataset with unequally spaced time intervals. In the latter, the first four measurements were performed with yearly intervals, while the fifth and sixth measurements were performed with 5-year intervals (Figure 1.1).

equally spaced time intervals

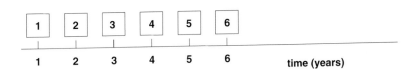

unequally spaced time intervals

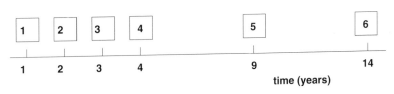

Figure 1.1. In the example dataset equally spaced time intervals and unequally spaced time intervals are used.

Table 1.2. Descriptive information[a] for an outcome variable Y and predictor variables X_1 to X_4[b] measured at six occasions

Time-point	Y	X_1	X_2	X_3	X_4
1	4.43 (0.67)	1.98 (0.22)	3.26 (1.24)	143/4	69/78
2	4.32 (0.67)	1.98 (0.22)	3.36 (1.34)	136/11	69/78
3	4.27 (0.71)	1.98 (0.22)	3.57 (1.46)	124/23	69/78
4	4.17 (0.70)	1.98 (0.22)	3.76 (1.50)	119/28	69/78
5	4.67 (0.78)	1.98 (0.22)	4.35 (1.68)	99/48	69/78
6	5.12 (0.92)	1.98 (0.22)	4.16 (1.61)	107/40	69/78

[a] For outcome variable Y and the continuous predictor variables (X_1 and X_2) mean and standard deviation are given, for the dichotomous predictor variables (X_3 and X_4) the numbers of subjects in the different categories are given.
[b] Y is serum cholesterol in mmol/l; X_1 is maximal oxygen uptake (in $(dl/min)/kg^{2/3}$); X_2 is the sum of four skinfolds (in cm); X_3 is smoking (non-smokers versus smokers); X_4 is gender (males versus females).

In the chapters dealing with dichotomous outcome variables, the continuous outcome variable Y is dichotomized (i.e. the highest tertile versus the other two tertiles) and in the chapter dealing with categorical outcome variables, the continuous outcome variable Y is divided into three equal groups (i.e. tertiles).

The dataset used in the examples is taken from the Amsterdam Growth and Health Study, an observational longitudinal study investigating the longitudinal relation between lifestyle and health in adolescence and young adulthood (Kemper, 1995). The abstract notation of the different variables (Y, X_1 to X_4) is used since it is basically unimportant what these variables actually are. The continuous outcome variable Y could be anything, a certain psychosocial variable (e.g. a score on a depression questionnaire, an indicator of quality of life, etc.) or a biological parameter (e.g. blood pressure, albumin concentration in blood, etc.). In this particular dataset the outcome variable Y was total serum cholesterol expressed in mmol/l. X_1 was fitness level at baseline (measured as maximal oxygen uptake on a treadmill), X_2 was body fatness (estimated by the sum of the thickness of four skinfolds), X_3 was smoking behaviour (dichotomized as smoking versus non-smoking) and X_4 was gender. Table 1.2 shows descriptive information for the variables used in the example.

1.5 Software

The relatively simple analyses of the example dataset were performed with SPSS (version 9; SPSS, 1997, 1998). For sophisticated longitudinal data analysis, other software packages were used. Generalized estimating equations (GEE) were performed with the Statistical Package for Interactive Data Analysis (SPIDA, version 6.05; Gebski et al., 1992). This statistical package is not often used, but the output is simple, and therefore very suitable for educational purposes. For random coefficient analysis STATA (version 7; STATA, 2001) was used. In Chapter 12, an overview (and comparison) will be given of other software packages such as SAS (version 8; Littel et al., 1991, 1996), S-PLUS (version 2000; Venables and Ripley, 1997; MathSoft, 2000), and MLwiN (version 1.02.0002; Goldstein et al., 1998; Rasbash et al., 1999). In all these packages algorithms to perform sophisticated longitudinal data analysis are implemented in the main software. Both syntax and output will accompany the overview of the different packages. For detailed information about the different software packages, reference is made to the software manuals.

1.6 Data structure

It is important to realize that different statistical software packages need different data structures in order to perform longitudinal analyses. In this respect a distinction must be made between a 'long' data structure and a 'broad' data structure. In the 'long' data structure each subject has as many data records as there are measurements over time, while in a 'broad' data structure each subject has one data record, irrespective of the number of measurements over time. SPSS for instance, uses a broad data structure, while SAS, MLwiN, S-PLUS, STATA and SPIDA use a 'long' data structure (Figure 1.2).

1.7 Statistical notation

The statistical notation will be very simple and straightforward. Difficult matrix notation will be avoided as much as possible. Throughout the book the number of subjects will be denoted as $i = 1$ to N, the number of times a

'long' data structure

ID	Y	time	X_4
1	3.5	1	1
1	3.7	2	1
1	3.9	3	1
1	3.0	4	1
1	3.2	5	1
1	3.2	6	1
2	4.1	1	1
2	4.1	2	1
.			
.			
N	5.0	5	2
N	4.7	6	2

'broad' data structure

ID	Y_{t1}	Y_{t2}	Y_{t3}	Y_{t4}	Y_{t5}	Y_{t6}	X_4
1	3.5	3.7	3.9	3.0	3.2	3.2	1
2	4.1	4.1	4.2	4.6	3.9	3.9	1
3	3.8	3.5	3.5	3.4	2.9	2.9	2
4	3.8	3.9	3.8	3.8	3.7	3.7	1
.							
.							
N	4.0	4.6	4.7	4.3	4.7	5.0	2

Figure 1.2. Illustration of two different data structures.

certain individual is measured will be denoted as $t = 1$ to T, and the number of predictor variables will be noted as $j = 1$ to J. Furthermore, the outcome variable will be called Y, and the predictor variables will be called X. All other notations will be explained below the equations where they are used.

Study design

2.1 Introduction

Epidemiological studies can be roughly divided into observational and experimental studies (see Figure 2.1). Observational studies can be further divided into case–control studies and cohort studies. Case–control studies are never longitudinal, in the way that longitudinal studies were defined in Chapter 1. The outcome variable Y (a dichotomous outcome variable distinguishing 'case' from 'control') is measured only once. Furthermore, case–control studies are always retrospective in design. The outcome variable Y is observed at a certain time-point, and the possible predictors are measured retrospectively.

In general, cohort studies can be divided into prospective, retrospective and cross-sectional cohort studies. A prospective cohort study is the only cohort study that can be characterized as a longitudinal study. Cohort studies are usually designed to analyse the longitudinal development of a certain characteristic over time. It is argued that this longitudinal development concerns growth processes. However, in studies investigating the elderly, the process of deterioration is the focus of the study, whereas in other developmental processes growth and deterioration can alternately follow each other. Moreover, in many epidemiological studies one is interested not only in the actual growth or deterioration over time, but also in the relationship between the developments of several characteristics over time. In these studies, the research question to be addressed is whether an increase (or decrease) in a certain outcome variable Y is associated with an increase (or decrease) in one or more predictor variables (X). Another important aspect of epidemiological observational prospective studies is that sometimes one is not really interested in growth or deterioration, but rather in the 'stability' of a certain characteristic over time. In epidemiology this phenomenon is known as tracking (see Chapter 11).

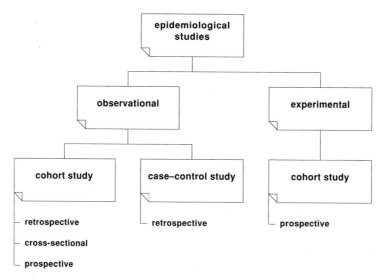

Figure 2.1. Schematic illustration of different epidemiological study designs.

Experimental studies, which in epidemiology are often referred to as clinical trials, are by definition prospective, i.e. longitudinal. The outcome variable Y is measured at least twice (the classical 'pre-test', 'post-test' design), and other intermediate measures are usually also added to the research design (e.g. to evaluate short-term and long-term effects). The aim of an experimental (longitudinal) study is to analyse the effect of one or more interventions on a certain outcome variable Y.

In Chapter 1, it was mentioned that some misunderstanding exists with regard to causality in longitudinal studies. However, an experimental study or clinical trial is basically the only epidemiological study design in which the issue of causality can be covered. With observational longitudinal studies, on the other hand, the question of probable causality remains unanswered.

Most of the statistical techniques in the examples covered in this book will be illustrated with data from an observational longitudinal study. In a separate chapter (Chapter 9), examples from experimental longitudinal studies will be discussed extensively. Although the distinction between experimental and observational longitudinal studies is obvious, in most situations the statistical techniques discussed for observational longitudinal studies are also suitable for experimental longitudinal studies.

2.2 Observational longitudinal studies

In observational longitudinal studies investigating individual development, each measurement taken on a subject at a particular time-point is influenced by three factors: (1) age (time from date of birth to date of measurement), (2) period (time or moment at which the measurement is taken), and (3) birth cohort (group of subjects born in the same year). When studying individual development, one is mainly interested in the age effect. One of the problems of most of the designs used in studies of development is that the main age effect cannot be distinguished from the two other 'confounding' effects (i.e. period and cohort effects).

2.2.1 Period and cohort effects

There is an extensive amount of literature describing age, period and cohort effects (e.g. Lebowitz, 1996; Robertson et al., 1999). However, most of the literature deals with classical age–period–cohort models, which are used to describe and analyse trends in (disease-specific) morbidity and mortality (e.g. Kupper et al., 1985; Mayer and Huinink, 1990; Holford, 1992; McNally et al., 1997; Robertson and Boyle, 1998). In this book, the main interests are the individual development over time, and the 'longitudinal' relationship between different variables. In this respect, period effects or time of measurement effects are often related to a change in measurement method over time, or to specific environmental conditions at a particular time of measurement. An example is given in Figure 2.2. This figure shows the longitudinal development of physical activity with age. Physical activity patterns were measured with a five-year interval, and were measured during the summer in order to minimize seasonal influences. The first measurement was taken during a summer with normal weather conditions. During the summer when the second measurement was taken, the weather conditions were extremely good, resulting in activity levels that were very high. At the time of the third measurement the weather conditions were comparable to the weather conditions at the first measurement, and therefore the physical activity levels were much lower than those recorded at the second measurement. When all the results are presented in a graph, it is obvious that the observed age trend is highly biased by the 'period' effect at the second measurement.

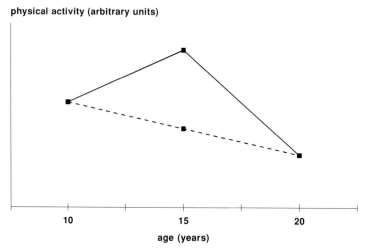

Figure 2.2. Illustration of a possible time of measurement effect (– – – 'real' age trend, ——— observed age trend).

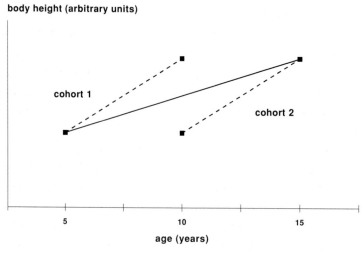

Figure 2.3. Illustration of a possible cohort effect (– – – cohort specific, ——— observed).

One of the most striking examples of a cohort effect is the development of body height with age. There is an increase in body height with age, but this increase is highly influenced by the increase in height of the birth cohort. This phenomenon is illustrated in Figure 2.3. In this hypothetical study, two repeated measurements were carried out in two different cohorts. The purpose of the study was to detect the age trend in body height. The first

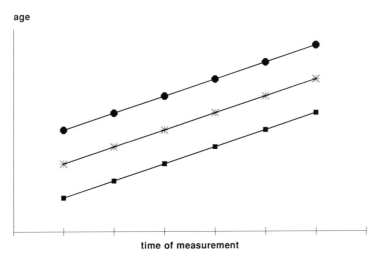

Figure 2.4. Principle of a multiple longitudinal design; repeated measurements of different cohorts with overlapping ages (■ cohort 1, ∗ cohort 2, • cohort 3).

cohort had an initial age of 5 years; the second cohort had an initial age of 10 years. At the age of 5, only the first cohort was measured, at the age of 10, both cohorts were measured, and at the age of 15 only the second cohort was measured. The body height obtained at the age of 10 is the average value of the two cohorts. Combining all measurements in order to detect an age trend will lead to a much flatter age trend than the age trends observed in both cohorts separately.

Both cohort and period effects can have a dramatic influence on interpretation of the results of longitudinal studies. An additional problem is that it is very difficult to disentangle the two types of effects. They can easily occur together. Logical considerations regarding the type of variable of interest can give some insight into the plausibility of either a cohort or a period effect. When there are (confounding) cohort or period effects in a longitudinal study, one should be very careful with the interpretation of age-related results.

It is sometimes argued that the design that is most suitable for studying individual growth/deterioration processes is a so-called 'multiple longitudinal design'. In such a design the repeated measurements are taken in more than one cohort with overlapping ages (Figure 2.4). With a 'multiple longitudinal design' the main age effect can be distinguished from cohort and period effects. Because subjects of the same age are measured at different time-points, the difference in outcome variable Y between subjects of the

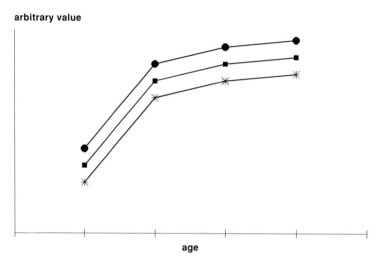

arbitrary value

age

Figure 2.5. Possibility of detecting cohort effects in a 'multiple longitudinal design' (∗ cohort 1, ▪ cohort 2, • cohort 3).

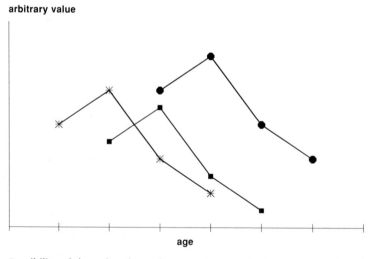

arbitrary value

age

Figure 2.6. Possibility of detecting time of measurement effects in a 'multiple longitudinal design' (∗ cohort 1, ▪ cohort 2, • cohort 3).

same age, but measured at different time-points, can be investigated in order to detect cohort effects. Figure 2.5 illustrates this possibility: different cohorts have different values at the same age.

Because the different cohorts are measured at the same time-points, it is also possible to detect possible time of measurement effects in a 'multiple longitudinal design'. Figure 2.6 illustrates this phenomenon. All three cohorts

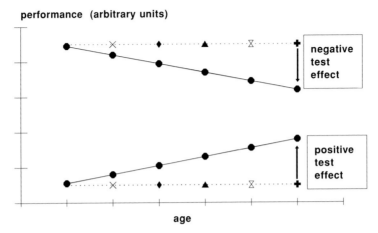

Figure 2.7. Test or learning effects; comparison of repeated measurements of the same subjects with non-repeated measurements in comparable subjects (different symbols indicate different subjects, ⋯⋯ cross-sectional, —— longitudinal).

show an increase in the outcome variable at the second measurement, which indicates a possible time of measurement effect.

2.2.2 Other confounding effects

In studies investigating development, in which repeated measurements of the same subjects are performed, cohort and period effects are not the only possible confounding effects. The individual measurements can also be influenced by a changing attitude towards the measurement itself, a so-called test or learning effect. This test or learning effect, which is illustrated in Figure 2.7, can be either positive or negative.

One of the most striking examples of a positive test effect is the measurement of memory in older subjects. It is assumed that with increasing age, memory decreases. However, even when the time interval between subsequent measurements is as long as three years, an **increase** in memory performance with increasing age can be observed: an increase which is totally due to a learning effect (Dik et al., 2001).

Furthermore, missing data or drop-outs during follow-up can have important implications for the interpretation of the results of longitudinal data analysis. This important issue will be discussed in detail in Chapter 10.

Analysis based on repeated measurements of the same subject can also be biased by a low degree of reproducibility of the measurement itself. This is quite important because the changes over time within one subject can be 'overruled' by a low reproducibility of the measurements. An indication of reproducibility can be provided by analysing the inter-period correlation coefficients (IPC) (van 't Hof and Kowalski, 1979). It is assumed that the IPCs can be approximated by a linear function of the time interval. The IPC will decrease as the time interval between the two measurements under consideration increases. The intercept of the linear regression line between the IPC and the time interval can be interpreted as the instantaneous measurement–remeasurement reproducibility (i.e. the correlation coefficient with a time interval of zero). Unfortunately, there are a few shortcomings in this approach. For instance, a linear relationship between the IPC and the time interval is assumed, and it is questionable whether that is the case in every situation. When the number of repeated measurements is low, the regression line between the IPC and the time interval is based on only a few data points, which makes the estimation of this line rather unreliable. Furthermore, there are no objective rules for the interpretation of this reproducibility coefficient. However, it must be taken into account that low reproducibility of measurements can seriously influence the results of longitudinal analysis.

2.2.3 Example

Table 2.1 shows the inter-period correlation coefficients (IPC) for outcome variable Y in the example dataset. To obtain a value for the measurement–remeasurement reproducibility, a linear regression analysis between the length of the time interval and the IPCs was carried out. The value of the intercept of that particular regression line can be seen as the IPC for a time interval with a length of zero, and can therefore be interpreted as a reproducibility coefficient (Figure 2.8).

The result of the regression analysis shows an intercept of 0.81, i.e. the reproducibility coefficient of outcome variable Y is 0.81. It has already been mentioned that it is difficult to provide an objective interpretation of this coefficient. Another important issue is that the interpretation of the coefficient highly depends on the explained variance (R^2) of the regression line (which is 0.67 in this example). In general, the lower the explained variance of the regression line, the more variation in IPCs with the same time interval, and the less reliable the estimation of the reproducibility coefficient.

Table 2.1. Inter-period correlation coefficients (IPC) for outcome variable Y

	Y_{t1}	Y_{t2}	Y_{t3}	Y_{t4}	Y_{t5}	Y_{t6}
Y_{t1}	—	0.76	0.70	0.67	0.64	0.59
Y_{t2}		—	0.77	0.78	0.67	0.59
Y_{t3}			—	0.85	0.71	0.63
Y_{t4}				—	0.74	0.65
Y_{t5}					—	0.69
Y_{t6}						—

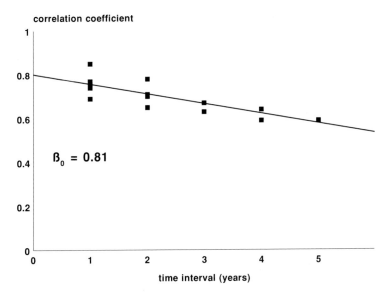

Figure 2.8. Linear regression line between the inter-period correlation coefficients and the length of the time interval.

2.3 Experimental (longitudinal) studies

Experimental (longitudinal) studies are by definition prospective cohort studies. A distinction can be made between randomized and non-randomized experimental studies. In epidemiology, randomized experimental studies are often referred to as randomized clinical trials (RCTs). In randomized experimental studies the subjects are randomly assigned to the experiment, i.e. intervention (or interventions) under study. The main reason for this

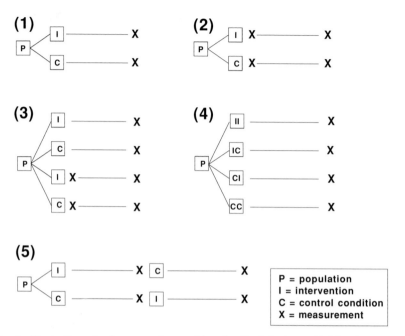

Figure 2.9. An illustration of a few experimental longitudinal designs: (1) 'classic' experimental design, (2) 'classic' experimental design with baseline measurement, (3) 'Solomon four group' design, (4) factorial design and (5) 'cross-over' design.

randomization is to make the groups to be compared as equal as possible at the start of the intervention.

It is not the purpose of this book to give a detailed description of all possible experimental designs. Figure 2.9 summarizes a few commonly used experimental designs. For an extensive overview of this topic, reference is made to other books (e.g. Pockok, 1983; Judd et al., 1991; Rothman and Greenland, 1998).

In the classical randomized experimental design, the population under study is randomly divided into an intervention group and a non-intervention group (e.g. a placebo group or a group with 'usual' care, etc.). The groups are then measured after a certain period of time to investigate the differences between the groups in the outcome variable. Usually, however, a baseline measurement is performed before the start of the intervention. The so-called 'Solomon four group' design is a combination of the design with and without a baseline measurement. The idea behind this design is that when a baseline measurement is performed there is a possibility of test or learning effects, and with a 'Solomon four group' design these test or learning effects can be detected. In a factorial design, two or more interventions are combined into one experimental study.

In the experimental designs discussed before, the subjects are randomly assigned to two or more groups. In studies of this type, basically all subjects have missing data for all other conditions, except the intervention to which they have been assigned. In contrast, it is also possible that all of the subjects are assigned to all possible interventions, but that the sequence of the different interventions is randomly assigned to the subjects. Experimental studies of this type are known as 'cross-over trials'. They are very efficient and very powerful, but they can only be performed for short-lasting outcome measures.

Basically, all the 'confounding' effects described for observational longitudinal studies (Section 2.2) can also occur in experimental studies. In particular, missing data or drop-outs are a major problem in experimental studies (see Chapter 10). Test or learning effects can be present, but cohort and time of measurement effects are less likely to occur.

It has already been mentioned that for the analysis of data from experimental studies all techniques that will be discussed in the following chapters, with examples from an observational longitudinal study, can also be used. However, Chapters 8 and 9 especially will provide useful information regarding the data analysis of experimental studies.

Continuous outcome variables

3.1 Two measurements

The simplest form of longitudinal study is that in which a continuous outcome variable Y is measured twice in time (Figure 3.1). With this simple longitudinal design the following question can be answered: 'Does the outcome variable Y change over time?' Or, in other words: 'Is there a difference in the outcome variable Y between t_1 and t_2?'

To obtain an answer to this question, a paired t-test can be used. Consider the hypothetical dataset presented in Table 3.1. The paired t-test is used to test the hypothesis that the mean difference between Y_{t1} and Y_{t2} equals zero. Because the **individual** differences are used in this statistical test, it takes into account the fact that the observations within one individual are dependent on each other. The test statistic of the paired t-test is the average of the differences divided by the standard deviation of the differences divided by the square root of the number of subjects (Equation (3.1)).

$$t = \frac{\bar{d}}{\left(\frac{s_d}{\sqrt{N}}\right)} \tag{3.1}$$

where t is the test statistic, $\bar{d}$ is the average of the differences, s_d is the standard deviation of the differences, and N is the number of subjects.

This test statistic follows a t-distribution with $(N-1)$ degrees of freedom. The assumptions for using the paired t-test are twofold, namely (1) that the observations of **different** subjects are independent and (2) that the differences between the two measurements are approximately normally distributed. In research situations in which the number of subjects is quite large (say above 25), the paired t-test can be used without any problems. With smaller datasets, however, the assumption of normality becomes important. When the assumption is violated, the non-parametric equivalent of the

Table 3.1. Hypothetical dataset for a longitudinal study with two measurements

i	Y_{t1}	Y_{t2}	Difference (d)
1	3.5	3.7	−0.2
2	4.1	4.1	0.0
3	3.8	3.5	0.3
4	3.8	3.9	−0.1
⋮			
N	4.0	4.6	−0.6

arbitrary value

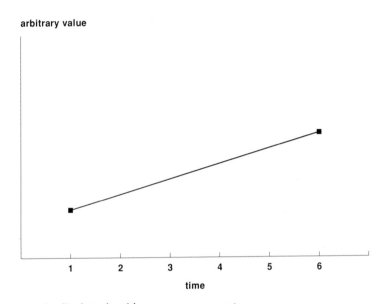

time

Figure 3.1. Longitudinal study with two measurements.

paired t-test can be used (see Section 3.2). In contrast to its non-parametric equivalent, the paired t-test is not only a testing procedure. With this statistical technique the average of the paired differences with the corresponding 95% confidence interval can also be estimated.

It should be noted that when the differences are not normally distributed and the sample size is rather large, the paired t-test provides valid results, but interpretation of the average differences can be complicated, because the average is not a good indicator of the mid-point of the distribution.

3.1.1 Example

One of the limitations of the paired t-test is that the technique is only suitable for two measurements over time. It has already been mentioned that the example dataset used throughout this book consists of six measurements. To illustrate the paired t-test in the example dataset, only the first and last measurements of this dataset are used. The question to be answered is: 'Is there a difference in outcome variable Y between $t = 1$ and $t = 6$?' Output 3.1 shows the results of the paired t-test.

Output 3.1. Results of a paired t-test performed on the example dataset

```
t-Tests for Paired Samples
              Number of              2-tail
Variable pairs      Corr     Sig          Mean     SD     SE of Mean
YT1 OUTCOME VARIABLE Y AT T1             4.4347   0.674  0.056
            147         0.586    0.000
YT6 OUTCOME VARIABLE Y AT T6             5.1216   0.924  0.076

Paired Differences
Mean                      SD     SE of Mean  t-value  df    2-tail Sig
-0.6869                   0.760  0.063       -10.96   146   0.000
95% CI      (-0.811,  -0.563)
```

The first lines of the output give descriptive information (i.e. mean values, standard deviation (SD), number of pairs, etc.), which is not really important in the light of the postulated question. The second part of the output provides the more important information. First of all, the mean of the paired differences is given (i.e. −0.6869), and also the 95% confidence interval (CI) around this mean (−0.811 to −0.563). A negative value indicates that there is an increase in outcome variable Y between $t = 1$ and $t = 6$. Furthermore, the results of the actual paired t-test are given: the value of the test statistic ($t = -10.96$), with $(N - 1)$ degrees of freedom (146), and the corresponding p-value (0.000). The results indicate that the increase in outcome variable Y is statistically significant ($p < 0.001$). The fact that there is a significant increase over time was already clear in the 95% confidence interval of the mean difference, which did not include zero.

Table 3.2. Hypothetical dataset for a longitudinal study with two measurements

i	Y_{t1}	Y_{t2}	Difference (d)	Rank number
1	3.5	3.7	−0.2	3
2	4.1	4.0	0.1	1.5[a]
3	3.8	3.5	0.3	4
4	3.8	3.9	−0.1	1.5[a]
5	4.0	4.4	−0.4	5
6	4.1	4.9	−0.8	7
7	4.0	3.4	0.6	6
8	5.1	6.8	−1.7	9
9	3.7	6.3	−2.6	10
10	4.1	5.2	−1.1	8

[a] The average rank is used for tied values.

3.2 Non-parametric equivalent of the paired *t*-test

When the assumptions of the paired *t*-test are violated, it is possible to perform the non-parametric equivalent of the paired *t*-test, the (Wilcoxon) signed rank sum test. This signed rank sum test is based on the ranking of the individual difference scores, and does not make any assumptions about the distribution of the outcome variable. Consider the hypothetical dataset presented in Table 3.2. The dataset consists of 10 subjects, who were measured on two occasions.

The signed rank sum test evaluates whether the sum of the rank numbers with a positive difference is equal to the sum of the rank numbers with a negative difference. When those two are equal, it suggests that there is no change over time. In the hypothetical dataset the sum of the rank numbers with a positive difference is 11.5 (i.e. $1.5 + 4 + 6$), while the sum of the rank numbers with a negative difference is 43.5. The exact calculation of the level of significance is very complicated, and goes beyond the scope of this book. All statistical handbooks contain tables in which the level of significance can be found (see for instance Altman, 1991), and with all statistical software packages the levels of significance can be calculated. For the hypothetical example, the *p*-value is between 0.2 and 0.1, indicating no significant change over time.

The (Wilcoxon) signed rank sum test can be used in all longitudinal studies with two measurements. It is a testing technique which only provides p-values, without effect estimation. In 'real life' situations, it will only be used when the sample size is very small (i.e. less than 25).

3.2.1 Example

Although the sample size in the example dataset is large enough to perform a paired t-test, in order to illustrate the technique the (Wilcoxon) signed rank sum test will be used to test whether or not the difference between Y at $t = 1$ and Y at $t = 6$ is significant. Output 3.2 shows the results of this analysis.

Output 3.2. Output of the (Wilcoxon) matched pairs signed rank sum test

```
Wilcoxon Matched-pairs Signed-ranks Test
       YT1      OUTCOME VARIABLE Y AT T1
   with YT6     OUTCOME VARIABLE Y AT T6


Mean Rank      Cases
    34.84        29      - Ranks     (YT6 Lt YT1)
    83.62        118     + Ranks     (YT6 Gt YT1)
                  0       Ties       (YT6 Eq YT1)
                 147      Total
 Z = -8.5637    2-tailed P = 0.0000
```

The first part of the output provides the mean rank of the rank numbers with a negative difference and the mean rank of the rank numbers with a positive difference. It also gives the number of cases with a negative and a positive difference. A negative difference corresponds with the situation that Y at $t = 6$ is less than Y at $t = 1$. This corresponds with a decrease in outcome variable Y over time. A positive difference corresponds with the situation that Y at $t = 6$ is greater than Y at $t = 1$, i.e. corresponds with an increase in Y over time. The last line of the output shows the Z-value. Although the (Wilcoxon) signed rank sum test is a non-parametric equivalent of the paired t-test, in many software packages a normal approximation is used to calculate the p-value. This Z-value corresponds with a highly significant p-value (0.0000), which indicates that there is a significant change (increase) over time in outcome variable Y. Because there is a **highly significant** change over time, the p-value obtained from the paired t-test is the same as the p-value obtained from the signed rank sum test. In general, however, the non-parametric tests are less powerful than the parametric equivalents.

3.3 More than two measurements

In a longitudinal study with more than two measurements performed on the same subjects (Figure 3.2), the situation becomes somewhat more complex. A design with only one outcome variable, which is measured several times on the same subjects, is known as a 'one-within' design. This refers to the fact that there is only one factor of interest (i.e. time) and that this factor varies only within individuals. In a situation with more than two repeated measurements, a paired t-test cannot be carried out. Consider the hypothetical dataset, which is presented in Table 3.3.

The question: 'Does the outcome variable Y change over time?' can be answered with multivariate analysis of variance (MANOVA) for repeated measurements. The basic idea behind this statistical technique is the same as for the paired t-test. The statistical test is carried out for the $T - 1$ absolute

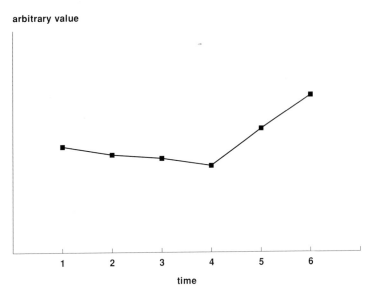

Figure 3.2. Longitudinal study with six measurements.

Table 3.3. Hypothetical dataset for a longitudinal study with more than two measurements

i	Y_{t1}	Y_{t2}	d_1	Y_{t3}	d_2	....	Y_{t6}	d_5
1	3.5	3.7	−0.2	3.9	−0.2		3.0	0.2
2	4.1	4.1	0.0	4.2	−0.1		4.6	0.0
3	3.8	3.5	0.3	3.5	0.0		3.4	−0.4
4	3.8	3.9	−0.1	3.8	0.1		3.8	0.3
⋮								
N	4.0	4.6	−0.6	4.7	−0.1		4.3	0.1

differences between subsequent measurements. In fact, MANOVA for repeated measurements is a multivariate analysis of these $T - 1$ absolute differences between subsequent time-points. Multivariate refers to the fact that $T - 1$ differences are used simultaneously as outcome variable. The $T - 1$ differences and corresponding variances and covariances form the test statistic for the MANOVA for repeated measurements (Equation (3.2)).

$$F = \left(\frac{N - T + 1}{(N - 1)(T - 1)} \right) H^2 \tag{3.2a}$$

$$H^2 = \frac{N y_d' y_d}{S_d^2} \tag{3.2b}$$

where F is the test statistic, N is the number of subjects, T is the number of repeated measurements, y_d' is the row vector of differences between subsequent measurements, y_d is the column vector of differences between subsequent measurements, and S_d^2 is the variance/covariance matrix of the differences between subsequent measurements.

The F-statistic follows an F-distribution with $(T - 1)$, $(N - T + 1)$ degrees of freedom. For a detailed description of how to calculate H^2 using Equation (3.2b), reference should be made to other textbooks (Crowder and Hand, 1990; Hand and Crowder, 1996; Stevens, 1996)[1]. As with all statistical techniques, MANOVA for repeated measurements is based on several

---

[1] H^2 is also known as Hotelling's T^2, and is often referred to as T^2. Because throughout this book T is used to denote the number of repeated measurements, H^2 is the preferred notation for this statistic.

assumptions. These assumptions are more or less comparable with the assumptions of a paired t-test: (1) observations of **different** subjects at each of the repeated measurements need to be independent, and (2) the observations need to be multivariate normally distributed, which is comparable but slightly more restrictive than the requirement that the differences between subsequent measurements be normally distributed. The calculation procedure described above is called the 'multivariate' approach because several differences are analysed together. However, to answer the same research question, a 'univariate' approach can also be followed. This 'univariate' procedure is comparable to the procedures carried out in simple analysis of variance (ANOVA) and is based on the 'sum of squares', i.e. squared differences between observed values and average values. The 'univariate' approach is only valid when, in addition to the earlier mentioned assumptions, an extra assumption is met: the assumption of 'sphericity'. This assumption is also known as the 'compound symmetry' assumption. It applies, firstly, when all correlations in outcome variable Y between repeated measurements are equal, irrespective of the time interval between the measurements. Secondly, the variances of outcome variable Y must be the same at each of the repeated measurements.

Whether or not the assumption of sphericity is met can be expressed by the sphericity coefficient (noted as ϵ). In an ideal situation the sphericity coefficient will equal one, and when the assumption is not entirely met, the coefficient will be less than one. In this case the degrees of freedom of the F-test used in the 'univariate' approach can be changed: instead of $(T-1)$, $(N-1)(T-1)$ the degrees of freedom will be $\epsilon(T-1)$, $\epsilon(N-1)(T-1)$. It should be noted that the degrees of freedom for the 'univariate' approach are different from the degrees of freedom for the 'multivariate' approach. In many software packages, when MANOVA for repeated measurements is carried out, the sphericity coefficient is automatically estimated and the degrees of freedom are automatically adapted. The sphericity coefficient can also be tested for significance (with the null hypotheses tested: sphericity coefficient $\epsilon = 1$). However, one must be very careful with the use of this test. If the sample size is large, the test for sphericity will (almost) always give a significant result, whereas in a study with a small sample size the test for sphericity will (almost) never give a significant result. In the first situation,

Table 3.4. Hypothetical longitudinal dataset with four measurements in six subjects

i	Y_{t1}	Y_{t2}	Y_{t3}	Y_{t4}	Mean
1	31	29	15	26	25.25
2	24	28	20	32	26.00
3	14	20	28	30	23.00
4	38	34	30	34	34.00
5	25	29	25	29	27.00
6	30	28	16	34	27.00
Mean	27.00	28.00	22.33	30.83	27.00

the test is over-powered, which means that even very small violations of the assumption of sphericity will be detected. In studies with small sample sizes, the test will be under-powered, i.e. the power to detect a violation of the assumption of sphericity is too low.

In the next section a numerical example will be given to explain the 'univariate' approach within MANOVA for repeated measurements.

3.3.1 The 'univariate' approach: a numerical example

Consider the simple longitudinal dataset presented in Table 3.4.

When ignoring the fact that **each individual** is measured four times, the question of whether there is a difference between the various time-points can be answered by applying a simple ANOVA, considering the measurements at the four time-points as four independent groups. The ANOVA is then based on a comparison between the 'between group' (in this case 'between time') sum of squares (SS_b) and the 'within group' (i.e. 'within time') sum of squares (SS_w). The latter is also known as the 'overall' sum of squares or the 'error' sum of squares. The sums of squares are calculated as follows:

$$SS_b = N \sum_{t=1}^{T} (\bar{y}_t - \bar{y})^2 \tag{3.3}$$

where N is the number of subjects, T is the number of repeated measurements, $\bar{y}_t$ is the average value of outcome variable Y at time-point t, and $\bar{y}$

is the overall average of outcome variable Y.

$$SS_w = \sum_{t=1}^{T} \sum_{n=1}^{N} (y_{it} - \bar{y}_t)^2 \tag{3.4}$$

where T is the number of repeated measurements, N is the number of subjects, y_{it} is the value of outcome variable Y for individual i at time-point t, and $\bar{y}_t$ is the average value of outcome variable Y at time-point t.

Applied to the dataset presented in Table 3.4, $SS_b = 6[(27 - 27)^2 + (28 - 27)^2 + (22.33 - 27)^2 + (30.83 - 27)^2] = 224.79$, and $SS_w = (31 - 27)^2 + (24 - 27)^2 + \cdots + (29 - 30.83)^2 + (34 - 30.83)^2 = 676.17$. These sums of squares are used in the ANOVA's F-test. In this test it is not the total sums of squares that are used, but the mean squares. The mean square (MS) is defined as the total sum of squares divided by the degrees of freedom. For SS_b, the degrees of freedom are $(T - 1)$, and for SS_w, the degrees of freedom are $(T) \times (N - 1)$. In the numerical example, $MS_b = 224.79/3 = 74.93$ and $MS_w = 676.17/20 = 33.81$. The F-statistic is equal to MS_b/MS_w and follows an F-distribution with $((T - 1), (T(N - 1))$ degrees of freedom. Applied to the example, the F-statistic is 2.216 with 3 and 20 degrees of freedom. The corresponding p-value (which can be found in a table of the F-distribution, available in all statistical textbooks) is 0.12, i.e. no significant difference between the four time-points. Output 3.3 shows the results of the ANOVA, applied to this numerical example.

Output 3.3. Results of an ANOVA with a simple longitudinal dataset, ignoring the dependency of observations

Source	Sum of squares	df	Mean square	F	Sig
Between groups	224.792	3	74.931	2.216	0.118
Within groups	676.167	20	33.808		
Total	900.958	23			

It has already been mentioned that in the above calculation the dependency of the observations was ignored. It was ignored that the **same** individual was measured four times. In a design with repeated measurements, the 'individual' sum of squares (SS_i) can be calculated (Equation (3.5)).

$$SS_i = T \sum_{i=1}^{N} (\bar{y}_i - \bar{y})^2 \tag{3.5}$$

where T is the number of repeated measurements, N is the number of subjects, $\bar{y}_i$ is the average value of outcome variable Y at all time-points for individual i, and $\bar{y}$ is the overall average of outcome variable Y.

Applied to the example dataset, $SS_i = 4[(25.25 - 27)^2 + (26 - 27)^2 + \cdots + (27 - 27)^2] = 276.21$. It can be seen that a certain proportion (276.21/676.17) of the error sum of squares (i.e. the within-time sum of squares) can be explained by individual differences. So, in this design with repeated measurements, the total error sum of squares of 676.17 is split into two components. The part which is due to individual differences (276.21) is now removed from the error sum of squares for the time effect. The latter is reduced to 399.96 (i.e. $676.17 - 276.21$). The SS_b is still the same, because this sum of squares reflects the differences between the four time-points. Output 3.4 shows the computer output of this example.

Output 3.4. Results of a MANOVA for repeated measurements with a simple longitudinal dataset

Within-subjects effects

Source	Sum of squares	df	Mean square	F	Sig
TIME	224.792	3	74.931	2.810	0.075
Error (TIME)	399.958	15	26.664		

Between-subjects effects

Source	Sum of squares	df	Mean square	F	Sig
Intercept	17550.042	1	17550.042	317.696	0.000
Error	276.208	5	55.242		

As mentioned before for the ANOVA, to carry out the F-test, the total sum of squares is divided by the degrees of freedom to create the 'mean square'. To obtain the appropriate F-statistic, the 'mean square' of a certain effect is divided by the 'mean square' of the error of that effect. The F-statistic is used in the testing procedure of that particular effect. As can be seen from Output 3.4, the SS_b is divided by $(T - 1)$ degrees of freedom, while the corresponding error term is divided by $(T - 1) \times (N - 1)$ degrees of freedom. The p-value is 0.075, which indicates no significant change over time. Note, however, that this p-value is somewhat lower than the p-value obtained from the simple ANOVA, in which the dependency of the observations was ignored. The intercept sum of squares is the sum of squares obtained when an overall average of zero is assumed. In this situation, the intercept sum of squares is useless, but it will be used in the analysis to investigate the shape of the relationship between the outcome variable Y and time.

3.3.2 The shape of the relationship between an outcome variable and time

In the foregoing sections of this chapter, the question of whether or not there is a change over time in outcome variable Y was answered. When such a change over time is found, this implies that there is some kind of relationship between the outcome variable Y and time. In this section the shape of the relationship between outcome variable Y and time will be investigated. In Figure 3.3 a few possible shapes are illustrated.

It is obvious that this question is only of interest when there are more than two measurements. When there are only two measurements, the only possible relationship with time is a linear one. The question about the shape of the relationship can also be answered by applying MANOVA for repeated measurements. In MANOVA, the relationship between the outcome variable Y and time is compared to a hypothetical linear relationship, a hypothetical quadratic relationship, and so on. When there are T repeated measurements, $T - 1$ possible functions with time can be tested. Although every possible

arbitrary value

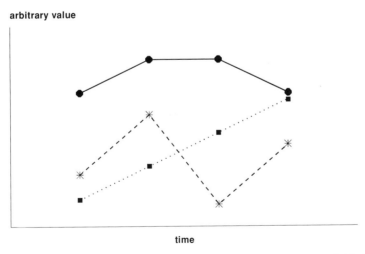

time

Figure 3.3. A few possible shapes of relationship between an outcome variable Y and time
(■······· linear, ●—— quadratic, ∗– – – cubic).

Table 3.5. Transformation 'factors' used to test different shapes of the relationship between an outcome variable and time

	Linear	Quadratic	Cubic
Y_{t1}	−0.671	0.500	−0.224
Y_{t2}	−0.224	−0.500	0.671
Y_{t3}	0.224	−0.500	−0.671
Y_{t4}	0.671	0.500	0.224

relationship with time can be tested, it is important to have a certain idea or hypothesis of the shape of the relationship between the outcome variable Y and time. It is highly recommended **not** to test all possible relationships routinely.

For each possible relationship, an F-statistic is calculated which follows an F-distribution with (1), $(N-1)$ degrees of freedom. The shape of the relationship between the outcome variable and time can only be analysed with the 'univariate' estimation approach. In the following section this will be illustrated with a numerical example.

3.3.3 A numerical example

Consider the same simple longitudinal dataset that was used in Section 3.3.1. To answer the question: 'What is the shape of the relationship between the outcome variable Y and time?', the outcome variable Y must be transformed. When there are four repeated measurements, Y is transformed into a linear component, a quadratic component and a cubic component. This transformation is made according to the transformation 'factors' presented in Table 3.5.

Each value of the original dataset is now multiplied by the corresponding transformation 'factor' to create a transformed dataset. Table 3.6 presents the linear transformed dataset. The asterisk above the name of a variable indicates that the variable is transformed.

These transformed variables are now used to test the different relationships with time. Assume that one is interested in the possible linear relationship with time. Therefore, the individual sum of squares for the linear transformed variables is related to the individual sum of squares calculated when the

Table 3.6. Original dataset transformed by linear transformation 'factors'

i	$Y_{t1}{}^{*}$	$Y_{t2}{}^{*}$	$Y_{t3}{}^{*}$	$Y_{t4}{}^{*}$	Mean
1	−20.8	−6.5	3.4	17.5	−1.62
2	−16.1	−6.3	4.5	21.5	0.89
3	−9.4	−4.5	6.3	20.1	3.13
4	−25.5	−7.6	6.7	22.8	−0.90
5	−16.8	−6.5	5.6	19.5	0.45
6	−20.1	−6.3	3.6	22.8	0.00
Mean					0.33

overall mean value of the transformed variables is assumed to be zero (i.e. the intercept).

The first step is to calculate the individual sum of squares for the transformed variables according to Equation (3.5). For the transformed dataset $\mathrm{SS_i}^{*} = 4[(-1.62 - 0.33)^2 + (0.89 - 0.33)^2 + \cdots + (0.00 - 0.33)^2] = 54.43$. The next step is to calculate the individual sum of squares when the overall mean value is assumed to be zero. When this calculation is performed for the transformed dataset $\mathrm{SS_i}^{0} = 4[(-1.62 - 0.00)^2 + (0.89 - 0.00)^2 + \cdots + (0.00 - 0.00)^2] = 56.96$.

The difference between these two individual sums of squares is called the 'intercept' and is shown in the computer output (see Output 3.5). In the example, this intercept is equal to 2.546, and this value is used to test for the linear development over time. The closer this difference comes to zero, the less likely it is that there is a linear relationship with time. In the example the p-value of the intercept is 0.65, which is far from significance, i.e. there is no significant linear relationship between the outcome variable and time.

Output 3.5. Results of MANOVA for repeated measurements, applied to the linear transformed dataset

```
Between-subjects effects
Source        Sum of squares   df   Mean square   F       Sig
Intercept     2.546            1    2.546         0.234   0.649
Error         54.425           5    10.885
```

When MANOVA for repeated measurements is performed on the original dataset used in Section 3.3.1, these transformations are automatically carried out and the related test values are shown on the output. Because the estimation procedure is slightly different to that explained here, the sums of squares given in this output are the sums of squares given in the output (see Output 3.6) multiplied by T. Because it is basically the same approach, the levels of significance are exactly the same.

Output 3.6. Results of MANOVA for repeated measurements, applied to the original dataset, analysing the linear relationship between the outcome variable and time

Within-subjects contrasts					
Source	Sum of squares	df	Mean square	F	Sig
Time(linear)	10.208	1	10.208	0.235	0.649
Error(linear)	217.442	5	43.488		

Exactly the same procedure can be carried out to test for a possible second-order (quadratic) relationship with time and for a possible third-order (cubic) relationship with time.

3.3.4 Example

The results of the MANOVA for repeated measurements of a 'one-within' design to answer the question of whether there is a change over time in outcome variable Y (using the information of all six repeated measurements) is shown in Output 3.7.

Output 3.7. Results of MANOVA for repeated measurements; a 'one-within' design

Multivariate tests[a]

Effect		Value	F	Hypothesis df	Error df	Sig	Partial Eta Squared
TIME	Pillai's Trace	0.666	56.615[b]	5.000	142.000	0.000	0.666
	Wilks'Lambda	0.334	56.615[b]	5.000	142.000	0.000	0.666
	Hotelling's Trace	1.993	56.615[b]	5.000	142.000	0.000	0.666
	Roy's Largest Root	1.993	56.615[b]	5.000	142.000	0.000	0.666

[a]Design: Intercept
Within subjects design: TIME
[b]Exact statistic.

Mauchly's test of sphericity[a]

Measure: MEASURE_1

| Within Subjects Effect | Mauchly's W | Approx. Chi-Square | df | Sig | Epsilon[b] | | |
					Greenhouse−Geisser	Huynh−Feldt	Lower-bound
TIME	0.435	119.961	14	0.000	0.741	0.763	0.200

Tests the null hypothesis that the error covariance matrix of the orthonormalized transformed dependent variables is proportional to an identity matrix.

[a]Design: Intercept

Within subjects design: TIME

[b]May be used to adjust the degrees of freedom for the averaged tests of significance. Corrected tests are displayed in the tests of within-subjects effects table.

Tests of within-subjects effects

Measure: MEASURE_1

Source		Type III Sum of Squares	df	Mean Square	F	Sig	Partial Eta Squared
TIME	Sphericity Assumed	89.987	5	17.997	99.987	0.000	0.406
	Greenhouse−Geisser	89.987	3.707	24.273	99.987	0.000	0.406
	Huynh−Feldt	89.987	3.816	23.582	99.987	0.000	0.406
	Lower-bound	89.987	1.000	89.987	99.987	0.000	0.406
Error (TIME)	Sphericity Assumed	131.398	730	0.180			
	Greenhouse−Geisser	131.398	541.272	0.243			
	Huynh−Feldt	131.398	557.126	0.236			
	Lower-bound	131.398	146.000	0.900			

Tests of within-subjects contrasts

Measure: MEASURE_1

Source	TIME	Type III Sum of Squares	df	Mean Square	F	Sig	Partial Eta Squared
TIME	Linear	40.332	1	40.332	126.240	0.000	0.464
	Quadratic	44.283	1	44.283	191.356	0.000	0.567
	Cubic	1.547	1	1.547	11.424	0.001	0.073
	Order 4	1.555	1	1.555	12.537	0.001	0.079
	Order 5	2.270	1	2.270	25.322	0.000	0.148
Error(TIME)	Linear	46.646	146	0.319			
	Quadratic	33.787	146	0.231			
	Cubic	19.770	146	0.135			
	Order 4	18.108	146	0.124			
	Order 5	13.088	146	8.964×10^{-2}			

The first part of the output (multivariate tests) shows directly the answer to the question of whether there is a change over time for outcome variable Y, somewhere between $t = 1$ and $t = 6$. The F-values and the significance levels are based on the multivariate test. In the output there are several multivariate tests available to test the overall time effect. The various tests are named after the statisticians who developed the tests, and they all use slightly different estimation procedures. However, the final conclusions of the various tests are almost always the same.

The second part of Output 3.7 provides information on whether or not the assumption of sphericity is met. In this example, the sphericity coefficient (epsilon) calculated by the Greenhouse–Geisser method is 0.741. The output also gives other values for ϵ (Huynh–Feldt and lower-bound), but these values are seldom used. The value of ϵ can be tested for significance by Mauchly's test of sphericity. The results of this test (p-value 0.000) indicates that ϵ is significantly different from the ideal value of one. This indicates that the degrees of freedom of the F-test should be adjusted. In the computer output presented, this correction is automatically carried out and is shown in the next part of the output (tests of within-subject effects), which shows the result of the 'univariate' estimation approach. The output of the 'univariate' approach gives four different estimates of the overall time effect. The first estimate is the one which assumes sphericity. The other three estimates (Greenhouse–Geisser, Huynh–Feldt and lower-bound) adjust for violations of the assumption of sphericity, by changing the degrees of freedom. The three techniques are slightly different, but it is recommended that the Greenhouse–Geisser adjustment is used, although this adjustment is slightly conservative. From the output it can be seen that the F-values and significance levels are equal for all estimation procedures. They are all highly significant, which indicates that there is a significant change over time in outcome variable Y. From the output, however, there is no indication of whether there is an increase, a decrease or whatever; it only shows a significant difference over time. Within MANOVA for repeated measurements, there is also the possibility to obtain a magnitude of the strength of the 'within-subject effect' (i.e. time). This magnitude is reflected in a measure called 'eta squared', which can be seen as an indicator for the explained variance in the outcome variable Y due to a particular effect.

Eta squared is calculated as the ratio between the sum of squares of the particular effect and the total sum of squares. From the output it can be seen that eta squared is 0.406 (i.e. 89.99/(131.40 + 89.99)), which indicates that 41% of the variance in outcome variable Y is explained by the time effect.

The last part of the output (tests of within-subjects contrasts) provides an answer to the second question ('what is the shape of the relationship with time?'). The first line (linear) indicates the test for a linear development. The F-value (obtained from the mean square (40.322) divided by the error mean square (0.319)) is very high (126.240), and is highly significant (0.000). This result indicates that there is a significant linear development over time. The following lines show the same values belonging to the other functions with time. The second line shows the second-order function (i.e. quadratic), the third line shows the third-order function (i.e. cubic), and so on. All F-values were significant, indicating that all other developments over time (second-order, third-order, etc.) are statistically significant. The magnitudes of the F-values, and the values of eta squared indicate further that the best way to describe the development over time is a quadratic function, but the more simple linear function with time is also quite good. Again, from the results there is no indication of whether there is an increase or a decrease over time. In fact, the results of the MANOVA for repeated measurements can only be interpreted correctly if a graphical representation of the change over time is made. Output 3.8 shows such a graphical representation. The figure shows that the significant development over time, which was found with MANOVA for repeated measurements, is first characterized by a small decrease, which is followed by an increase over time.

To put the results of the MANOVA for repeated measurements in a somewhat broader perspective, the results of a 'naive' analysis are shown in Output 3.9, naive in the sense that the dependency of the repeated observations within one subject is ignored. Such a naive analysis is an analysis of variance (ANOVA), in which the mean values of outcome variable Y are compared among all six measurements, i.e. six groups, each representing one time-point. For only two measurements, this comparison would be the same as the comparison between an independent sample t-test (the naive approach) and a paired t-test (the adjusted approach).

Output 3.8. Results of the MANOVA for repeated measurements; graphical representation of a 'one-within' design

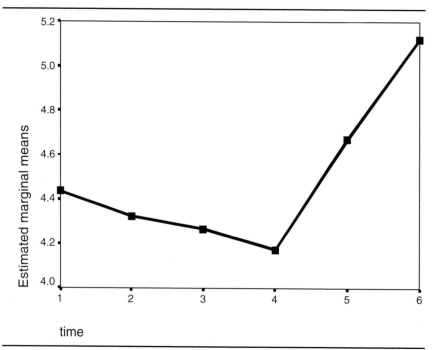

From Output 3.9 it can be seen that the F-statistic for the time effect (the effect in which we are interested) is 32.199, which is highly significant (0.000). This result indicates that at least one of the mean values of outcome variable Y at a certain time-point is significantly different from the mean value of outcome variable Y at one of the other time-points. However, as mentioned before, this approach ignores the fact that a longitudinal study is performed, i.e. that the same subjects are measured on several occasions. The most important difference between MANOVA for repeated measurements and the naive ANOVA is that the 'error sum of squares' in the ANOVA is much higher than the 'error sum of squares' in the MANOVA for repeated measurements. In the ANOVA this 'error sum of squares' (indicated by the residual mean square) is 0.559 (see Output 3.9), while for the MANOVA for repeated measurements this 'error sum of squares' (indicated by Error (TIME) Sphericity Assumed) was more than three times lower, i.e. 0.180 (see Output 3.7).

Output 3.9. Results of a (naive) analysis of variance (ANOVA), ignoring the dependency of observations

```
Analysis of Variance
            Y                    OUTCOME VARIABLE Y AT T1 TO T6
         BY TIME
                    Sum of              Mean              Signif
Source of Variation Squares   DF    Square    F          of F
Main Effects        89.987     5    17.997    32.199     0.000
TIME                89.987     5    17.997    32.199     0.000
Explained           89.987     5    17.997    32.199     0.000
Residual           489.630   876     0.559
Total              579.617   881     0.658
```

3.4 The 'univariate' or the 'multivariate' approach?

Within MANOVA for repeated measurements a distinction can be made between the 'multivariate' approach (the multivariate extension of a paired *t*-test) and the 'univariate' approach (an extension of ANOVA). The problem is that the two approaches do not produce the same results. So the question is: Which approach should be used?

One of the differences between the two approaches is the assumption of sphericity. For the 'multivariate' approach this assumption is not necessary, while for the 'univariate' approach it is an important assumption. The restriction of the assumption of sphericity (i.e. equal correlations and equal variances over time) leads to an increase in degrees of freedom, i.e. an increase in power for the 'univariate' approach. This increase in power becomes more important when the sample size becomes smaller. The 'multivariate' approach was developed later than the 'univariate' approach, especially for situations when the assumption of sphericity does not hold. So, one could argue that when the assumption of sphericity is violated, the 'multivariate' approach should be used. However, in the 'univariate' approach, adjustments can be made when the assumption of sphericity is not met. So, in principle, both approaches can deal with a situation in which the assumption of sphericity does not hold. It is sometimes argued that when the number of subjects N is less than the number of (repeated) measurements plus 10, the 'multivariate' approach should not be used. In every other situation, however, it is recommended that the results of both the 'multivariate' and the 'univariate' approach are used to obtain the most 'valid' answer to the research question addressed. Only when both approaches produce the same results, it is fairly certain that there is either a significant or a non-significant change over time. When both approaches produce different results, the conclusions must be drawn with many restrictions and considerable caution. In such a situation, it is highly recommended not to use the approach with the lowest p-value!

3.5 Comparing groups

In the first sections of this chapter longitudinal studies were discussed in which one continuous outcome variable is repeatedly measured over time (i.e. the 'one-within' design). In this section the research situation will be discussed in which the development of a certain continuous outcome variable Y is compared between different groups. This design is known as the 'one-within, one-between' design. Time is the within-subject factor and the group variable is the between-subjects factor (Figure 3.4). This group indicator can be either dichotomous or categorical. The question to be addressed is: 'Is there a difference in change over time for outcome variable Y between two or more groups?' This question can also be answered with MANOVA for repeated measurements. The same assumptions as have been mentioned

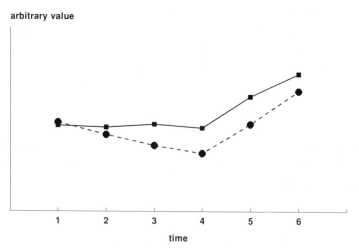

Figure 3.4. A longitudinal 'one-within, one-between' design with six repeated measurements measured in two groups (■—— group 1, ●– – – group 2).

earlier (Section 3.3) apply for this design, but it is also assumed that the covariance matrices of the different groups that are compared to each other are homogeneous. This assumption is comparable with the assumption of equal variances in two groups that are cross-sectionally compared with each other using the independent sample t-test. Although this is an important assumption, in reasonably large samples a violation of this assumption is generally not problematic.

From a 'one-within, one-between' design the following 'effects' can be obtained: (1) an overall time effect, i.e. 'is there a change over time in outcome variable Y for the total population?', (2) a general group effect, i.e. 'is there on average a difference in outcome variable Y between the compared groups?', (3) a group by time interaction effect, i.e. 'is the change over time in outcome variable Y different for the compared groups?' The within-subject effects can be calculated in two ways: the 'multivariate' approach, which is based on the multivariate analysis of the differences between subsequent points of measurements, and the 'univariate' approach, which is based on the comparison of several sums of squares (see Section 3.5.1). In epidemiological longitudinal studies the group by time interaction effect is probably the most interesting, because it gives an answer to the question of whether there is a difference in change over time between groups.

With respect to the shape of the relationship with time (linear, quadratic, etc.) specific questions can also be answered for the 'one-within, one-between' design, such as 'is there a difference in the linear relationship with time between the groups?', 'is there a difference in the quadratic relationship with time?', etc. However, especially for interaction terms, the answers to those questions can be quite complicated, i.e. the results of the MANOVA for repeated measurements can be very difficult to interpret.

It should be noted that an important limitation of MANOVA for repeated measurements is that the between-subjects factor can only be a time-independent dichotomous or categorical variable, such as treatment group, gender, etc.

3.5.1 The 'univariate' approach: a numerical example

The simple longitudinal dataset used to illustrate the 'univariate' approach in a 'one-within' design will also be used to illustrate the 'univariate' approach

Table 3.7. Hypothetical longitudinal dataset with four measurements in six subjects divided into two groups

i	Group	Y_{t1}	Y_{t2}	Y_{t3}	Y_{t4}	Mean
1	1	31	29	15	26	25.25
2	1	24	28	20	32	26.00
3	1	14	20	28	30	23.00
Mean		23.00	25.67	21.00	29.33	24.75
4	2	38	34	30	34	34.00
5	2	25	29	25	29	27.00
6	2	30	28	16	34	27.00
Mean		31.00	30.33	23.67	32.33	29.33

in a 'one-within, one-between' design. Therefore, the dataset used in the earlier example, and presented in Table 3.4, is extended to include a group indicator. The 'new' dataset is presented in Table 3.7.

To estimate the different 'effects', it should first be noted that part of the overall 'error sum of squares' is related to the differences between the two groups. To calculate this part, the sum of squares for individuals (SS_i) must be calculated for each of the groups (see Equation (3.5)). For group 1, $SS_i = 3[(25.25 - 24.75)^2 + (26 - 24.75)^2 + (23 - 24.75)^2] = 19.5$, and for group 2, $SS_i = 3[(34 - 29.33)^2 + (27 - 29.33)^2 + (27 - 29.33)^2] = 130.7$.

These two parts can be added together to give an overall 'error sum of squares' of 150.2. If the group indication is ignored, the overall 'error sum of squares' is 276.2 (see Section 3.3.1). This means that the between-subjects sum of squares caused by group differences is 126.0 (i.e. 276.2 − 150.2). The next step is to calculate the SS_w and the SS_b for each group. This can be done in the same way as has been described for the whole population (see Equations (3.3) and (3.4)). The results are summarized in Table 3.8.

The two within-subject 'error sums of squares' can be added together to form the overall within-subject error sum of squares (corrected for group). This total within-subject error sum of squares is 373.17. Without taking the group differentiation into account, a within-subject error sum of squares

Table 3.8. Summary of the different sums of squares calculated for each group separately

	Group 1	Group 2
SS_b	116.9	134.7
SS_w	299.3	224.0
SS_i	19.5	130.7
Within-subject error sum of squares	$299.3 - 19.5 = 279.83$	$224.0 - 130.7 = 93.33$

of 399.96 was found. The difference between the two is the sum of squares belonging to the interaction between the within-subject factor 'time' and the between-subject factor 'group'. This sum of squares is 26.79. Output 3.10 shows the computerized results of the MANOVA for repeated measurements for this numerical example.

Output 3.10. Results of MANOVA for repeated measurements for a simple longitudinal dataset with a group indicator

```
Within-subjects effects
Source          Sum of squares   df   Mean square   F       Sig
TIME            224.792           3   74.931        2.810   0.075
TIME × GROUP     26.792           3    8.931        0.287   0.834
Error(TIME)     373.167          12   31.097


Between-subjects effects
Source          Sum of squares   df   Mean square   F         Sig
Intercept       17550.042         1   17550.042     317.696   0.000
GROUP             126.042         1     126.042       3.357   0.141
Error             150.167         4      37.542
```

3.5.2 Example

In the example dataset, X_4 is a dichotomous time-independent predictor variable (i.e. gender), so this variable will be used as a between-subjects factor in this example. The results of the MANOVA for repeated measurements from a 'one-within, one-between' design are shown in Output 3.11.

Output 3.11. Results of MANOVA for repeated measurements; a 'one-within, one-between' design

Tests of between-subjects effects

Measure: MEASURE_1
Transformed Variable: Average

Source	Type III Sum of Squares	df	Mean Square	F	Sig	Partial Eta Squared
Intercept	17715.454	1	17715.454	7486.233	0.000	0.981
X4	15.103	1	15.103	6.382	0.013	0.042
Error	343.129	145	2.366			

Multivariate tests[a]

Effect		Value	F	Hypothesis df	Error df	Sig	Partial Eta Squared
TIME	Pillai's Trace	0.669	56.881[b]	5.000	141.000	0.000	0.669
	Wilks' Lambda	0.331	56.881[b]	5.000	141.000	0.000	0.669
	Hotelling's Trace	2.017	56.881[b]	5.000	141.000	0.000	0.669
	Roy's Largest Root	2.017	56.881[b]	5.000	141.000	0.000	0.669
TIME * X4	Pillai's Trace	0.242	8.980[b]	5.000	141.000	0.000	0.242
	Wilks' Lambda	0.758	8.980[b]	5.000	141.000	0.000	0.242
	Hotelling's Trace	0.318	8.980[b]	5.000	141.000	0.000	0.242
	Roy's Largest Root	0.318	8.980[b]	5.000	141.000	0.000	0.242

[a]Design: Intercept + X4
Within subjects design: TIME
[b]Exact statistic.

Mauchly's test of sphericity[a]

Measure: MEASURE_1

Within Subjects Effect	Mauchly's W	Approx. Chi-Square	df	Sig	Greenhouse –Geisser	Huynh–Feldt	Lower-bound
TIME	0.433	119.736	14	0.000	0.722	0.748	0.200

Epsilon[b] spans Greenhouse–Geisser, Huynh–Feldt, Lower-bound columns.

Tests the null hypothesis that the error covariance matrix of the orthonormalized transformed dependent variables is proportional to an identity matrix.
[a]Design: Intercept+X4
Within subjects design: TIME
[b]May be used to adjust the degrees of freedom for the averaged tests of significance. Corrected tests are displayed in the tests of within-subjects effects table.

Tests of within-subjects effects

Measure: MEASURE_1

Source		Type III Sum of Squares	df	Mean Square	F	Sig	Partial Eta Squared
TIME	Sphericity Assumed	89.546	5	17.909	104.344	0.000	0.418
	Greenhouse–Geisser	89.546	3.612	24.793	104.344	0.000	0.418
	Huynh–Feldt	89.546	3.741	23.937	104.344	0.000	0.418
	Lower-bound	89.546	1.000	89.546	104.344	0.000	0.418
TIME * X4	Sphericity Assumed	6.962	5	1.392	8.113	0.000	0.053
	Greenhouse–Geisser	6.962	3.612	1.928	8.113	0.000	0.053
	Huynh–Feldt	6.962	3.741	1.861	8.113	0.000	0.053
	Lower-bound	6.962	1.000	6.962	8.113	0.005	0.053
Error (TIME)	Sphericity Assumed	124.436	725	0.172			
	Greenhouse–Geisser	124.436	523.707	0.238			
	Huynh–Feldt	124.436	542.443	0.229			
	Lower-bound	124.436	145.000	0.858			

Tests of within-subjects contrasts

Measure: MEASURE_1

Source	TIME	Type III Sum of Squares	df	Mean Square	F	Sig	Partial Eta Squared
TIME	Linear	38.668	1	38.668	131.084	0.000	0.475
	Quadratic	45.502	1	45.502	213.307	0.000	0.595
	Cubic	1.602	1	1.602	11.838	0.001	0.075
	Order 4	1.562	1	1.562	12.516	0.001	0.079
	Order 5	2.212	1	2.212	24.645	0.000	0.145
TIME * X4	Linear	3.872	1	3.872	13.127	0.000	0.083
	Quadratic	2.856	1	2.856	13.388	0.000	0.085
	Cubic	0.154	1	0.154	1.142	0.287	0.008
	Order 4	7.533×10^{-3}	1	7.533×10^{-3}	0.060	0.806	0.000
	Order 5	7.216×10^{-2}	1	7.216×10^{-2}	0.804	0.371	0.006
Error (TIME)	Linear	42.773	145	0.295			
	Quadratic	30.931	145	0.213			
	Cubic	19.616	145	0.135			
	Order 4	18.100	145	0.125			
	Order 5	13.016	145	8.976×10^{-2}			

Part of the Output 3.11 is comparable to the output of the 'one-within' design, shown in Output 3.7. The major difference is found in the first part of the output, in which the result of the 'tests of between-subjects effects' is given. The F-value belonging to this test is 6.382 and the significance level is 0.013, which indicates that there is an overall (i.e. averaged over time) difference between the two groups indicated by X_4. The other difference between the two outputs is the addition of a time by X_4 (TIME* $X4$) interaction term. This interaction is interesting, because it answers the question of whether there is a difference in development over time between the two groups indicated by X_4 (i.e. the difference in developments between males and females). The answer to that question can either be obtained with the 'multivariate' approach (Pillai, Wilks, Hotelling, and Roy) or with the 'univariate' approach. For the 'multivariate' approach (multivariate tests), firstly the overall time effect is given and secondly the time by X_4 interaction. For the 'univariate' approach, again the assumption of sphericity has to hold and from the output it can be seen that this is not the case (Greenhouse–Geisser $\epsilon = 0.722$, and the significance of the sphericity test is 0.000). For this reason, in the univariate approach it is recommended that the Greenhouse–Geisser adjustment is used. From the output of the univariate analysis, firstly the overall time effect ($F = 104.344$, significance 0.000) and secondly the time by X_4 interaction effect ($F = 8.113$, significance 0.000) can be obtained. This result indicates that there is a significant difference in development over time between the two groups indicated by X_4.

From the next part of Output 3.11 (tests of within-subjects contrasts) it can be seen that this difference is significant for both the linear development over time and the quadratic development over time.

For all three effects, the explained variances are also given as an indicator of the magnitude of the effect. In this example it can be seen that 42% of the variance in outcome variable Y is explained by the 'time effect', that 5% is explained by the 'time by X_4 interaction', and that 4% of the variance in outcome variable Y is explained by the 'overall group effect'. Care must be taken in the interpretation of these explained variances, because they cannot be interpreted together in a straightforward way. The explained variances for the time effect and the time–group interaction effect are only related to the within-subject 'error sum of squares', and not to the total 'error sum of squares'.

As in the case for the 'one-within' design, the results of the MANOVA for repeated measurements for a 'one-within, one-between' design can only be interpreted correctly when a graphical representation is added to the results (see Output 3.12).

Output 3.12. Results of MANOVA for repeated measurements; graphical representation of a 'one-within, one-between' design (X_4, —— males, – – – females)

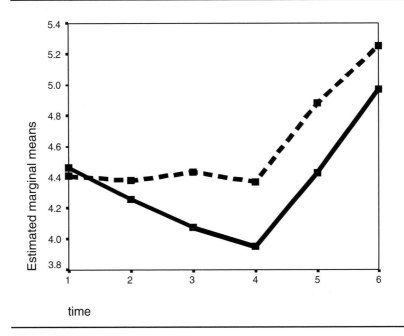

3.6 Comments

One of the problems with MANOVA for repeated measurements is that the time periods under consideration are weighted equally. A non-significant change over a short time period can be relatively greater than a significant change over a long time period. So, when the time periods are unequally spaced, the results of MANOVA for repeated measurements cannot be interpreted in a straightforward way. The length of the different time intervals must be taken into account.

Another major problem with MANOVA for repeated measurements is that it only takes into account the subjects with complete data, i.e. the subjects who are measured at all time-points. When a subject has no data available for a certain time-point, all other data for that subject are deleted from the analysis. In Chapter 10, the problems and consequences of missing data in longitudinal studies and in the results obtained from a MANOVA for repeated measurements analysis will be discussed. MANOVA for repeated measurements can also be used for more complex study designs, i.e. with more 'within-subject' and/or more 'between-subjects' factors. Because the ideas and the potential questions to be answered are the same as in the relatively simple designs discussed before, the more complex designs will not be discussed further. It should be kept in mind that the more groups that are compared to each other (given a certain number of subjects), or the more factors that are included in the design, the less power there will be to detect significant effects. This is important, because MANOVA for repeated measurements is basically a testing technique, so p-values are used to evaluate longitudinal relationships. In principle, no interesting effect estimations are provided by the procedure of the MANOVA for repeated measurements. The explained variances can be calculated, but the importance of this indicator is rather limited.

3.7 Post-hoc procedures

With MANOVA for repeated measurements an 'overall' time effect and an 'overall' group effect can be obtained. As in cross-sectional ANOVA, post-hoc procedures can be performed to investigate further the observed 'overall' relationships. In longitudinal analysis there are two types of these post-hoc procedures. (1) When there are more than two repeated measurements, it can be determined in which part of the longitudinal time period the observed 'effects' occur. This can be done by performing MANOVA for repeated measurements for a specific (shorter) time period. (2) When there are more than two groups for which the longitudinal relationship is analysed, a statistically significant 'between-subjects effect' indicates that there is a difference between at least two of the compared groups. Further analysis can determine between which groups the differences occur. This can be carried out by applying the post-hoc procedures also used in the cross-sectional ANOVA (e.g. Tukey procedure, Bonferroni procedure and Scheffe procedure). Each technique has is own particularities, but in essence multiple comparisons are made between all groups; each group is pairwise compared to the other groups.

3.7.1 Example

Output 3.13 shows a typical output of a post-hoc procedure following MANOVA for repeated measurements comparing three groups (the data are derived from a hypothetical dataset which will not be discussed any further).

Output 3.13. Results of three post-hoc procedures in MANOVA for repeated measurements

Between-subjects effects

Source	Sum of squares	df	Mean square	F	Sig
Intercept	17845.743	1	17845.743	8091.311	0.000
GROUP	40.364	2	20.317	9.221	0.000
Error	317.598	144	2.206		

Post-hoc tests

	Group1	Group2	Mean difference $(1 - 2)$	Std error	Sig
Tukey	1	2	-8.361×10^{-2}	0.1225	0.774
		3	-0.4913	0.1225	0.000
	2	1	-8.361×10^{-2}	0.1225	0.774
		3	-0.4077	0.1225	0.003
	3	1	0.4913	0.1225	0.000
		2	0.4077	0.1225	0.003
Scheffe	1	2	-8.361×10^{-2}	0.1225	0.793
		3	-0.4913	0.1225	0.000
	2	1	-8.361×10^{-2}	0.1225	0.793
		3	-0.4077	0.1225	0.005
	3	1	0.4913	0.1225	0.000
		2	0.4077	0.1225	0.005
Bonferroni	1	2	-8.361×10^{-2}	0.1225	1.00
		3	-0.4913	0.1225	0.000
	2	1	-8.361×10^{-2}	0.1225	1.00
		3	-0.4077	0.1225	0.003
	3	1	0.4913	0.1225	0.000
		2	0.4077	0.1225	0.003

The structure of the first part of the output is similar to the outputs discussed before. It shows the overall between-subjects group effect. The p-value belonging to this group effect is highly significant. The interpretation of this result is that there is at least one significant difference between two of the three groups, but this overall result gives no information about which groups actually differ from each other. To obtain an answer to that question, a post-hoc procedure can be carried out. In the output, the results of the three most commonly used post-hoc procedures are given. The first column of the output gives the name of the post-hoc procedure (Tukey, Scheffe and Bonferroni). The second and third columns show the pairwise comparisons that are made, and the fourth and fifth columns give the overall mean difference between the compared groups and the standard error of that difference. The last column gives the p-value of the pairwise comparison. One must realize that these post-hoc procedures deal with the **overall** between-subjects group effect, i.e. the difference between the average value over the different time-points. To obtain an answer to the question in which part of the longitudinal period the observed relationships occurred, a MANOVA can be performed for specific time periods.

As can be seen from the output, there are only marginal differences between the three post-hoc procedures (in most research situations this will be the case). It can be seen that groups 1 and 2 do not differ from each other, but that the average value of group 3 is totally different from that of the other two groups.

3.8 Different contrasts

In an earlier part of this chapter, attention was paid to answering the question: 'What is the shape of the relationship between outcome variable Y and time?' In the example it was mentioned that the answer to that question can be found in the output section: test of within-subject contrasts. In the example a so-called 'polynomial' contrast was used in order to investigate whether one is dealing with a linear relationship with time, a quadratic relationship with time, and so on. In longitudinal research this is by far the most important contrast, but there are many other possible contrasts (depending on the software package used). With a 'simple' contrast, for instance, the value at each measurement is related to the first measurement.

With a 'difference' contrast, the value of each measurement is compared to the average of all **previous** measurements. A 'Helmert' contrast is comparable to the 'difference' contrast, however, the value at a particular measurement is compared to the average of all **subsequent** measurements. With the 'repeated' contrast, the value of each measurement is compared to the value of the first subsequent measurement. In Section 3.3 it was mentioned that the testing of a 'polynomial' contrast was based on transformed variables. In fact, the testing of all contrasts is based on transformed variables. However, for each contrast, different transformation coefficients are used.

3.8.1 Example

Outputs 3.14a to 3.14d show the results of MANOVA for repeated measurements with different contrasts performed on the example dataset. The output obtained from the analysis with a polynomial contrast was already shown in Section 3.4 (Output 3.7).

With the 'simple' contrast, each measurement is compared to the first measurement. From Output 3.14a it can be seen that all follow-up measurements differ significantly from the first measurement. From the output, however, it cannot be seen whether the value at $t = 2$ is higher than the value at $t = 1$. It can only be concluded that there is a significant difference.

With the 'difference' contrast, the value at each measurement is compared to the average value of all previous measurements. From Output 3.14b it can be seen that there is a significant difference between the value at each measurement and the average value of all previous measurements.

With the 'Helmert' contrast (Output 3.14c), the same procedure is carried out as with the 'difference' contrast, only the other way around. The value at each measurement is compared to the average value of all subsequent measurements. All these differences are also highly significant. Only if we compare the first measurement with the average value of the other five measurements, is the p-value of borderline significance (0.047).

With the 'repeated' contrast, the value of each measurement is compared to the value of the first subsequent measurement. From Output 3.14d it can be seen that the value of outcome variable Y at $t = 2$ is not significantly different to the value of outcome variable Y at $t = 3$ ($p = 0.136$). All the other differences investigated were statistically significant. Again, it must be stressed that there is no information about whether the value at a particular time-point is higher or lower than the value at the first subsequent time-point. Like all other results obtained from MANOVA for repeated measurements, the results of the analysis with different contrasts can only be interpreted correctly if they are combined with a graphical representation of the development of outcome variable Y.

Output 3.14a. Results of MANOVA for repeated measurements with a 'simple' contrast

```
Within-subject Contrasts
Source               Sum of squares   df  Mean square  F          Sig
Level2 vs Level1     1.830            1   1.830          8.345    0.004
Level3 vs Level1     4.184            1   4.184         14.792    0.000
Level4 vs Level1    10.031            1  10.031         32.096    0.000
Level5 vs Level1     8.139            1   8.139         20.629    0.000
Level6 vs Level1    69.353            1  69.353        120.144    0.000
Error
Level2 vs Level1    32.010          146   0.219
Level3 vs Level1    41.296          146   0.283
Level4 vs Level1    45.629          146   0.313
Level5 vs Level1    57.606          146   0.395
Level6 vs Level1    84.279          146   0.577
```

Output 3.14b. Results of MANOVA for repeated measurements with a 'difference' contrast

```
Within-subject Contrasts
Source                Sum of squares   df  Mean square  F          Sig
Level1 vs Level2       1.830           1   1.830          8.345    0.004
Level2 vs Previous     1.875           1   1.875          9.679    0.002
Level3 vs Previous     4.139           1   4.139         28.639    0.000
Level4 vs Previous    20.198           1  20.198         79.380    0.000
Level5 vs Previous    82.271           1  82.271        196.280    0.000
Error
Level1 vs Level2      32.010         146   0.219
Level2 vs Previous    28.260         146   0.194
Level3 vs Previous    21.101         146   0.145
Level4 vs Previous    37.150         146   0.254
Level5 vs Previous    61.196         146   0.419
```

Output 3.14c. Results of MANOVA for repeated measurements with a 'Helmert' contrast

```
Within-subject Contrasts
Source               Sum of squares   df  Mean square   F         Sig
Level1 vs Later      0.852             1   0.852           4.005   0.047
Level2 vs Later      8.092             1   8.092          41.189   0.000
Level3 vs Later     22.247             1  22.247         113.533   0.000
Level4 vs Later     76.695             1  76.695         277.405   0.000
Level5 vs Level6    29.975             1  29.975          63.983   0.000
Error
Level1 vs Later     31.061          146   0.213
Level2 vs Later     28.684          146   0.196
Level3 vs Later     28.609          146   0.196
Level4 vs Later     40.365          146   0.276
Level5 vs Level6    68.399          146   0.468
```

Output 3.14d. Results of MANOVA for repeated measurements with a 'repeated' contrast

```
Within-subject Contrasts
Source               Sum of squares   df  Mean square   F         Sig
Level1 vs Level2     1.830            1   1.830           8.345   0.004
Level2 vs Level3     0.480            1   0.480           2.242   0.136
Level3 vs Level4     1.258            1   1.258           8.282   0.005
Level4 vs Level5    36.242            1  36.242         125.877   0.000
Level5 vs Level6    29.975            1  29.975          63.983   0.000
Error
Level1 vs Level2    32.010         146   0.219
Level2 vs Level3    31.260         146   0.214
Level3 vs Level4    22.182         146   0.152
Level4 vs Level5    42.036         146   0.288
Level5 vs Level6    68.399         146   0.468
```

When there are more than two groups to be compared with MANOVA for repeated measurements, contrasts can also be used to perform post-hoc procedures for the 'overall' group effect. With the traditional post-hoc procedures discussed in Section 3.7 all groups are pairwise compared, while with contrasts this is not the case. With a 'simple' contrast for instance, the groups are compared to a certain reference category, and with a 'repeated' contrast each group is compared to the next group (dependent on the coding of the group variable). The advantage of contrasts in performing post-hoc procedures is when a correction for certain covariates is applied. In that situation, the traditional post-hoc procedures cannot be performed, while with contrasts, the **adjusted** difference between groups can be obtained. Again, it is important to realize that the post-hoc procedures performed with different contrasts are only suitable (as the traditional post-hoc procedures) for analysing the 'between-subjects' effect.

3.9 Non-parametric equivalent of MANOVA for repeated measurements

When the assumptions of MANOVA for repeated measurements are violated, an alternative non-parametric approach can be applied. This non-parametric equivalent of MANOVA for repeated measurements is called the Friedman test and can only be used in a 'one-within' design. Like any other non-parametric test, the Friedman test does not make any assumptions about the distribution of the outcome variable under study. To perform the Friedman test, for each subject the outcome variable at T time-points is ranked from 1 to T. The Friedman test statistic is based on these rankings. In fact, the mean rankings (averaged over all subjects) at each time-point are compared to each other. The idea behind the Friedman test is that the observed rankings are compared to the expected rankings, assuming there is no change over time. The Friedman test statistic can be calculated according to Equation (3.6):

$$H = \frac{12 \sum_{t=1}^{T} R_t^2}{NT(T+1)} - 3N(T+1) \tag{3.6}$$

where H is the Friedman test statistic, R_t is the sum of the ranks at time-point t, N is the number of subjects, and T is the number of repeated measurements.

To illustrate this non-parametric test, consider again the hypothetical dataset presented earlier in Table 3.4. In Table 3.9 the ranks of this dataset

Table 3.9. Absolute values and ranks (in parentheses) of the hypothetical dataset presented in Table 3.4

i	Y_{t1} (rank)	Y_{t2} (rank)	Y_{t3} (rank)	Y_{t4} (rank)
1	31 (4)	29 (3)	15 (1)	26 (2)
2	24 (2)	28 (3)	20 (1)	32 (4)
3	14 (1)	20 (2)	28 (3)	30 (4)
4	38 (4)	34 (2.5)	30 (1)	34 (2.5)
5	25 (1.5)	29 (3.5)	25 (1.5)	29 (3.5)
6	30 (3)	28 (2)	16 (1)	34 (4)
Total rank	15.5	16	8.5	20

are presented. Applied to the (simple) longitudinal dataset the Friedman test statistic (H) is equal to:

$$\frac{12(15.5^2 + 16^2 + 8.5^2 + 20^2)}{6 \times 4 \times 5} - 3 \times 6 \times 5 = 6.85$$

This value follows a χ^2 distribution with $T - 1$ degrees of freedom. The corresponding p-value is 0.077. When this p-value is compared to the value obtained from a MANOVA for repeated measurements (see Output 3.4) it can be seen that they are almost the same. That the p-value from the non-parametric test is slightly higher than the p-value from the parametric test has to do with the fact that non-parametric tests are in general less powerful than the parametric equivalents.

3.9.1 Example

Because the number of subjects in the example dataset is reasonably high, in practice the Friedman test will not be used in this situation. However, for educational purposes the non-parametric Friedman test will be used to answer the question of whether there is a development over time in outcome variable Y. Output 3.15 shows the results of this analysis.

From the output it can be seen that there is a significant difference between the measurements at different time-points. The χ^2 statistic is 244.1535, and with five degrees of freedom (the number of measurements minus

Output 3.15. Output of the non-parametric Friedman test

```
Friedman Two-way ANOVA
Mean Rank    Variable
3.49         YT1          OUTCOME VARIABLE Y AT T1
2.93         YT2          OUTCOME VARIABLE Y AT T2
2.79         YT3          OUTCOME VARIABLE Y AT T3
2.32         YT4          OUTCOME VARIABLE Y AT T4
4.23         YT5          OUTCOME VARIABLE Y AT T5
5.24         YT6          OUTCOME VARIABLE Y AT T6
Cases        Chi-Square   DF    Significance
147          244.1535     5     0.0000
```

one) this value is highly significant, i.e. a similar result to that found with the MANOVA for repeated measurements. The Friedman test statistic gives no direct information about the direction of the development, although from the mean rankings it can be seen that a decrease from the second to the fourth measurement is followed by an increase at the fifth and sixth measurements.

Continuous outcome variables – relationships with other variables

4.1 Introduction

With a paired t-test and MANOVA for repeated measurements it is possible to investigate changes in one continuous variable over time and to compare the development of a continuous variable over time between different groups. These methods, however, are not suitable for analysis of the relationship between the developments of two continuous variables or for analysis of the relationship between a continuous outcome variable and several predictor variables, which can be either continuous, dichotomous or categorical. Before the development of 'sophisticated' statistical techniques such as generalized estimating equations (GEE) and random coefficient analysis, 'traditional' methods were used to analyse longitudinal data. The general idea of these 'traditional' methods was to reduce the statistical longitudinal problem into a cross-sectional problem. Even nowadays these (limited) approaches are often used in the analysis of longitudinal data.

4.2 'Traditional' methods

The greatest advantage of the 'traditional' methods is that simple cross-sectional statistical techniques can be used to analyse the longitudinal data. The most commonly used technique for reducing the longitudinal problem to a cross-sectional problem is analysis of the relationships between changes in different parameters between two points in time (Figure 4.1). Because of its importance and its widespread use, a detailed discussion of the analysis of changes is given in Chapter 8.

Another traditional method with which to analyse the longitudinal relationship between several variables is the use of a single measurement at the end of the longitudinal period as outcome variable. This outcome variable is

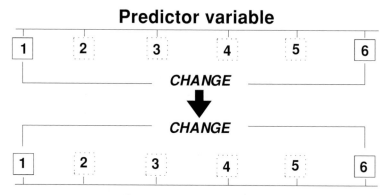

Figure 4.1. Changes in outcome variable *Y* between two subsequent measurements are related to changes in one or more predictor variable(s) *X* over the same time period.

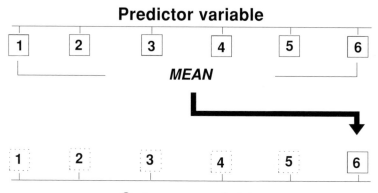

Figure 4.2. 'Long-term exposure' to one or more predictor variable(s) *X* related to a single measurement of outcome variable *Y*.

then related to a so-called 'long-term exposure' to certain predictor variables, measured along the total longitudinal period (Figure 4.2).

It is obvious that a limitation of both methods is that if there are more than two measurements, not all available longitudinal data are used in the analysis. Another cross-sectional possibility for analysing the longitudinal relationship between an outcome variable *Y* and (several) predictor variables *X*, using all the data, is to use individual regression lines with time. The first step in this procedure is to calculate the linear regression between the outcome variable Y and time for each subject. The regression coefficient with time (which is referred to as the slope) can be seen as an indicator for the change over the whole measurement period in the outcome variable Y. This regression coefficient with time is then used as the outcome variable in a cross-sectional regression analysis, in order to investigate the longitudinal relationship with other variables. The same procedure can be followed for the time-dependent predictor variables in order to analyse the relationship between the change in outcome variable Y and the change in the time-dependent predictor variables. However, the baseline value of the predictor variables can also be used in the final cross-sectional regression analysis. In the latter case it is obvious that a different research question is answered. The greatest disadvantage of this technique is the assumption of a linear relationship between the outcome variable Y and time, although it is possible to model a different individual regression function with time. Furthermore, it is questionable how well the individual regression line (or function), which is usually based on a few data points, fits the observed data.

4.3 Example

To illustrate the first 'cross-sectional' technique that can be used to analyse the longitudinal relationship between a continuous outcome variable Y and several predictor variables X (Figure 4.1), the change between Y_{t1} and Y_{t6} is first calculated. In the next step the changes in the time-dependent predictor variables X_2 and X_3 must be calculated. For X_3, which is a dichotomous predictor variable, this is rather difficult, because the interpretation of the changes is not straightforward. In Chapter 8 this problem will be discussed further. In this example, the subjects were divided (according to X_3) into subjects who remained in the lowest category or 'decreased' between $t = 1$ and $t = 6$ (i.e. the non-smokers and the subjects who quitted smoking), and subjects who remained in the highest category or 'increased' between $t = 1$ and $t = 6$ (i.e. the ever-smokers and the subjects who started to smoke). Because the longitudinal problem is reduced into a cross-sectional problem, the relationships can be analysed with simple linear regression analysis. The result of the analysis is shown in Output 4.1.

Because the longitudinal problem is reduced to a cross-sectional problem, and the data are analysed with simple cross-sectional regression analysis, the regression coefficient can be interpreted in a straightforward way. For

Output 4.1. Results of a linear regression analysis relating changes in predictor variables to changes in outcome variable Y between $t=1$ and $t=6$

	B	Std. error	Standardized coefficient	t	Sig
Constant	-0.140	0.851		-0.165	0.870
X1	0.127	0.348	0.037	0.364	0.716
DELX2	0.046	0.044	0.087	1.055	0.293
DELX3	-0.051	0.141	-0.030	-0.364	0.716
X4	0.359	0.153	0.236	2.341	0.021

Dependent variable: DELY

instance, the regression coefficient for X_4 indicates that the difference between Y at $t=1$ and Y at $t=6$ is 0.359 higher for the group indicated by $X_4 = 2$ (i.e. females) compared to the group indicated by $X_4 = 1$ (i.e. males).

The second cross-sectional technique is slightly different. In this method 'long-term exposure' to the predictor variables X is related to the outcome variable Y at $t=6$ (Figure 4.2). For the time-dependent predictor variable X_2, the average of the six measurements was used as indicator for 'long-term exposure'. For the dichotomous predictor variable X_3, the 'long-term exposure' is coded as 0 when subjects report 0 (i.e. non-smoking) at all measurements, and coded 1 when subjects report 1 (i.e. smoking) at least at one of the measurements. The result of the linear regression analysis is shown in Output 4.2.

Output 4.2. Results of a linear regression analysis relating 'long-term exposure' to predictor variables to the outcome variable Y at $t=6$

	B	Std. error	Standardized coefficient	t	Sig
Constant	2.380	1.027		2.317	0.022
X1	0.719	0.407	0.171	1.768	0.079
AveragX2	0.373	0.068	0.518	5.495	0.000
AveragX3	0.085	0.141	0.046	0.605	0.546
X4	-0.073	0.182	-0.040	-0.405	0.686

Dependent variable: OUTCOME VARIABLE Y AT T6

The output shows for instance a highly significant relationship between the average value of X_2 (calculated over all six repeated measurements) and the outcome variable Y at $t = 6$; a relationship which can be interpreted in such a way that a 1 point higher 'long-term exposure' to X_2 is associated with a 0.373 point higher value for Y at $t = 6$.

The last mentioned cross-sectional method that can be used to analyse a longitudinal relationship is based on the individual linear regression lines between outcome variable Y and time. The individual regression coefficients with time (i.e. the slopes) are then used as outcome variable in a linear regression analysis relating the development of outcome variable Y to several predictor variables. It has already been mentioned that the predictor variables can be modelled in many different ways, depending on the research question at issue. In this example the relationship between the values of all predictor variables at $t = 1$ and the slopes of the individual regression lines of outcome variable Y was investigated, in order to obtain an answer to the question of whether or not the development in outcome variable Y can be predicted by predictor variables measured at baseline. The result of this analysis is shown in Output 4.3.

Output 4.3. Results of a linear regression analysis relating baseline values of the predictor variables to the slopes of the individual regression lines between outcome variable Y and time

	B	Std. error	Standardized coefficient	t	Sig
Constant	-0.159	0.158		-1.002	0.318
X1	0.051	0.063	0.084	0.824	0.411
X2	0.026	0.010	0.247	2.684	0.008
X3	-0.021	0.067	-0.026	-0.328	0.743
X4	0.063	0.026	0.235	2.418	0.017

Dependent variable: SLOPEY

In this analysis, both X_2 (measured at baseline) and X_4 are significantly and positively related to the linear increase in the outcome variable Y between $t = 1$ and $t = 6$. Subjects with $X_4 = 2$ (i.e. females) have a 0.063 higher slope than the subjects with $X_4 = 1$ (i.e. males). The way the 'slope' has to be interpreted depends on the way time is modelled. Because in the example dataset the outcome variable Y is measured at yearly intervals, the slope of the linear regression with time can be interpreted as the yearly increase in outcome variable Y.

So far, three relatively simple analyses have been performed to investigate the 'longitudinal' relationship between the outcome variable Y and the four predictor variables X. It should be stressed that although all three analyses were based on the same dataset, and were performed to determine the longitudinal relationship between outcome variable Y and the four predictor variables X, the different analyses produce different results. It should be realized that longitudinal relationships can be very complicated, and that different types of analysis should be performed to investigate different aspects of longitudinal relationships.

4.4 Longitudinal methods

With the development of (new) statistical techniques, such as GEE and random coefficient analysis, it has become possible to analyse longitudinal relationships using all available longitudinal data, without summarizing the longitudinal development of each subject into one value. The longitudinal relationship between a continuous outcome variable Y and one or more predictor variable(s) X (Figure 4.3) can be described by Equation (4.1).

$$Y_{it} = \beta_0 + \sum_{j=1}^{J} \beta_{1j} X_{itj} + \varepsilon_{it} \tag{4.1}$$

where Y_{it} are observations for subject i at time t, β_0 is the intercept, X_{ijt} is the independent variable j for subject i at time t, β_{1j} is the regression coefficient for independent variable j, J is the number of independent variables, and ε_{it} is the 'error' for subject i at time t.

This model is almost the same as a cross-sectional linear regression model, except for the subscripts t. These subscripts indicate that the outcome variable Y is repeatedly measured on the same subject (i.e. the definition of a longitudinal study), and that the predictor variable X can be repeatedly measured on the same subject. In this model the coefficients of interest are β_{1j}, because these regression coefficients show the magnitude of the relationship between the longitudinal development of the outcome variable (Y_{it}) and

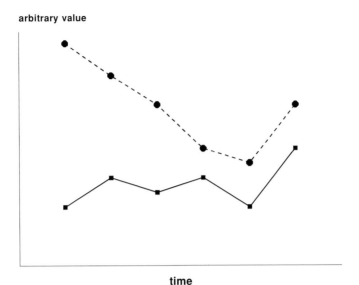

arbitrary value

time

Figure 4.3. Longitudinal relationship between outcome variable Y and predictor variable X
(■ —— outcome variable, • – – – predictor variable).

the development of the predictor variables (X_{ijt}). The first extension to this model is the addition of a time indicator t (Equation (4.2)).

$$Y_{it} = \beta_0 + \sum_{j=1}^{J} \beta_{1j} X_{itj} + \beta_2 t + \varepsilon_{it} \tag{4.2}$$

where Y_{it} are observations for subject i at time t, β_0 is the intercept, X_{ijt} is the independent variable j for subject i at time t, β_{1j} is the regression coefficient for independent variable j, J is the number of independent variables, t is time, β_2 is the regression coefficient for time, and ε_{it} is the 'error' for subject i at time t.

This simple model can be extended to a general form, in which a correction for both time-dependent covariates (Z_{ikt}) and time-independent covariates (G_{im}) is modelled (Equation (4.3)).

$$Y_{it} = \beta_0 + \sum_{j=1}^{J} \beta_{1j} X_{itj} + \beta_2 t + \sum_{k=1}^{K} \beta_{3k} Z_{ikt} + \sum_{m=1}^{M} \beta_{4m} G_{im} + \varepsilon_{it} \tag{4.3}$$

where Y_{it} are observations for subject i at time t, β_0 is the intercept, X_{ijt} is the independent variable j for subject i at time t, β_{1j} is the regression coefficient for independent variable j, J is the number of independent variables,

t is time, β_2 is the regression coefficient for time, Z_{ikt} is the time-dependent covariate k for subject i at time t, β_{3k} is the regression coefficient for time-dependent covariate k, K is the number of time-dependent covariates, G_{im} is the time-independent covariate m for subject i, β_{4m} is the regression coefficient for time-independent covariate m, M is the number of time-independent covariates, and ε_{it} is the 'error' for subject i at time t.

In this general model, again the coefficients of interest are β_{1j}, because these regression coefficients express the relationships between the longitudinal development of the outcome variable (Y_{it}) and the development of different predictor variables (X_{ijt}). Predictor variables and covariates can be either continuous, dichotomous or categorical. For the latter, the same procedure as in cross-sectional linear regression analyses has to be followed, i.e. dummy variables must be created for each of the categories. In the following sections two sophisticated methods (GEE and random coefficient analysis) will be discussed. Both techniques are highly suitable for estimation of the regression coefficients of the general model given in Equation (4.3).

4.5 Generalized estimating equations

4.5.1 Introduction

With GEE the relationships between the variables of the model at different time-points are analysed simultaneously. So, the estimated β_1 reflects the relationship between the longitudinal development of the outcome variable Y and the longitudinal development of corresponding predictor variables X, using all available longitudinal data (Figure 4.3). GEE is an iterative procedure, using quasi-likelihood to estimate the regression coefficients (Liang and Zeger, 1986; Zeger and Liang, 1986; Zeger et al., 1988; Zeger and Liang, 1992; Liang and Zeger, 1993; Lipsitz et al., 1994a). The details of quasi-likelihood will not be discussed. An extensive explanation of quasi-likelihood can be found in several other publications (McCullagh, 1983; Nelder and Pregibon, 1987; Zeger and Qaqish, 1988; Nelder and Lee, 1992; Diggle et al., 1994).

4.5.2 Working correlation structures

Because the repeated observations within one subject are not independent of each other, a correction must be made for these within-subject correlations. With GEE, this correction is carried out by assuming a priori a certain 'working' correlation structure for the repeated measurements of the outcome variable Y. Depending on the software package used to estimate the regression coefficients, there is a choice between various correlation structures. The first possibility is an **independent structure**. With this structure the correlations between subsequent measurements are assumed to be zero. In fact, this option is counterintuitive because a special technique is being used to correct for the dependency of the observations and this correlation structure assumes independence of the observations:

	t_1	t_2	t_3	t_4	t_5	t_6
t_1	—	0	0	0	0	0
t_2	0	—	0	0	0	0
t_3	0	0	—	0	0	0
t_4	0	0	0	—	0	0
t_5	0	0	0	0	—	0
t_6	0	0	0	0	0	—

A second possible choice for a working correlation structure is an **exchangeable structure**. In this structure the correlations between subsequent measurements are assumed to be the same, irrespective of the length of the time interval:

	t_1	t_2	t_3	t_4	t_5	t_6
t_1	—	ρ	ρ	ρ	ρ	ρ
t_2	ρ	—	ρ	ρ	ρ	ρ
t_3	ρ	ρ	—	ρ	ρ	ρ
t_4	ρ	ρ	ρ	—	ρ	ρ
t_5	ρ	ρ	ρ	ρ	—	ρ
t_6	ρ	ρ	ρ	ρ	ρ	—

A third possible working correlation structure, the so-called (**stationary**) m-**dependent structure** assumes that the correlations t measurements apart are equal, the correlations $t + 1$ measurements apart are assumed to be equal, and so on for $t = 1$ to $t = m$. Correlations more than m measurements apart are assumed to be zero. When, for instance, a '2-dependent correlation structure' is assumed, all correlations one measurement apart are assumed to be the same, all correlations two measurements apart are assumed to be the same, and the correlations more than two measurements apart are assumed to be zero:

	t_1	t_2	t_3	t_4	t_5	t_6
t_1	—	ρ_1	ρ_2	0	0	0
t_2	ρ_1	—	ρ_1	ρ_2	0	0
t_3	ρ_2	ρ_1	—	ρ_1	ρ_2	0
t_4	0	ρ_2	ρ_1	—	ρ_1	ρ_2
t_5	0	0	ρ_2	ρ_1	—	ρ_1
t_6	0	0	0	ρ_2	ρ_1	—

A fourth possibility is an **autoregressive correlation structure**, i.e. the correlations one measurement apart are assumed to be ρ; correlations two measurements apart are assumed to be ρ^2; correlations t measurements apart are assumed to be ρ^t.

	t_1	t_2	t_3	t_4	t_5	t_6
t_1	—	ρ^1	ρ^2	ρ^3	ρ^4	ρ^5
t_2	ρ^1	—	ρ^1	ρ^2	ρ^3	ρ^4
t_3	ρ^2	ρ^1	—	ρ^1	ρ^2	ρ^3
t_4	ρ^3	ρ^2	ρ^1	—	ρ^1	ρ^2
t_5	ρ^4	ρ^3	ρ^2	ρ^1	—	ρ^1
t_6	ρ^5	ρ^4	ρ^3	ρ^2	ρ^1	—

The least restrictive correlation structure, is the **unstructured correlation structure**. With this structure, all correlations are assumed to be different:

	t_1	t_2	t_3	t_4	t_5	t_6
t_1	—	ρ_1	ρ_2	ρ_3	ρ_4	ρ_5
t_2	ρ_1	—	ρ_6	ρ_7	ρ_8	ρ_9
t_3	ρ_2	ρ_6	—	ρ_{10}	ρ_{11}	ρ_{12}
t_4	ρ_3	ρ_7	ρ_{10}	—	ρ_{13}	ρ_{14}
t_5	ρ_4	ρ_8	ρ_{11}	ρ_{13}	—	ρ_{15}
t_6	ρ_5	ρ_9	ρ_{12}	ρ_{14}	ρ_{15}	—

In the literature it is assumed that GEE analysis is robust against a wrong choice of correlation matrix (i.e. it does not matter much which correlation structure is chosen, the results of the longitudinal analysis will be more or less the same) (Liang and Zeger, 1986; Zeger and Liang, 1986). However, when the results of analyses with different working correlation structures are compared to each other, they differ in such a way that they can lead to 'wrong' conclusions about longitudinal relationships between several variables (Twisk et al., 1997). It is therefore important to realize which correlation structure is most appropriate for the analysis. Unfortunately, with GEE there is no straightforward way to determine which correlation structure should be used. One of the possibilities is to analyse the within-subject correlation structure of the observed data to find out which possible structure is the best approximation of the 'real' correlation structure[1]. Furthermore, the simplicity of the correlation structure has to be taken into account when choosing a certain working correlation structure. The number of parameters (in this case correlation coefficients) that need to be estimated differs for each of the various working correlation structures. For instance, for an exchangeable structure only one correlation coefficient has to be estimated, while for a stationary 5-dependent structure, five correlation coefficients must be estimated. Assuming an unstructured correlation structure in a longitudinal study with six repeated measurements, 15 correlation coefficients must be estimated. As a result, the power of the statistical analysis is influenced by the choice of a certain structure. Basically, the best choice is the simplest correlation structure which fits the data well.

In order to enhance insight in GEE analysis, the estimation procedure can be seen as follows. First a 'naive' linear regression analysis is carried out, assuming the observations within subjects are independent. Then, based on the residuals of this analysis, the parameters of the working correlation matrix are calculated. The last step is to re-estimate the regression coefficients, correcting for the dependency of the observations. Although the whole procedure is slightly more complicated (i.e. the estimation process alternates between steps two and three, until the estimates of the regression coefficients and standard errors stabilize), it basically consists of the three above-mentioned steps (see Burton et al., 1998).

In GEE analysis, the within-subject correlation structure is treated as a 'nuisance' variable (i.e. as a covariate). So, in principle, the way in which GEE analysis corrects for the dependency of observations within one subject is the way that has been shown in Equation (4.4) (which can be seen as an extension of Equation (4.3)).

$$Y_{it} = \beta_0 + \sum_{j=1}^{J} \beta_{1j} X_{itj} + \beta_2 t + \cdots + \text{CORR}_{it} + \varepsilon_{it} \tag{4.4}$$

---

[1] One must realize that, in fact, GEE corrects for correlated errors (ε_{it} in Equations (4.1) to (4.3)). The correlated errors are caused by the correlated observations, but they are not exactly the same. Adding predictor variables to the longitudinal model, for instance, can lead to another correlation structure in the errors than the one approximated by the within-subject correlation structure of the observed data.

where Y_{it} are observations for subject i at time t, β_0 is the intercept, X_{ijt} is the independent variable j for subject i at time t, β_{1j} is the regression coefficient for independent variable j, J is the number of independent variables, t is time, β_2 is the regression coefficient for time, CORR_{it} is the working correlation structure, and ε_{it} is the 'error' for subject i at time t.

4.5.3 Interpretation of the regression coefficients derived from GEE analysis

Basically, the regression coefficient β_1 for a particular predictor variable relates the 'vector' of outcomes over time to the 'vector' of the predictor variable over time:

$$
\begin{bmatrix} Y_1 \\ Y_2 \\ Y_3 \\ Y_4 \\ Y_5 \\ Y_6 \end{bmatrix} = \beta_0 + \beta_1 \begin{bmatrix} X_1 \\ X_2 \\ X_3 \\ X_4 \\ X_5 \\ X_6 \end{bmatrix} + \cdots
$$

Unfortunately, there is no simple straightforward interpretation of the regression coefficient β_1. In fact, GEE analysis based on the model presented here includes a 'pooled' analysis of longitudinal and cross-sectional relationships; or in other words, it combines a **within-subject** relationship with a **between-subjects** relationship, resulting in one single regression coefficient. This has the following implications for interpretation of the regression coefficients. Suppose that for a particular subject the value of an outcome variable Y is relatively high at each of the repeated measurements, and that this value does not change much over time. Suppose further that for that particular subject the value of a particular predictor variable X is also relatively high at each of the repeated measurements, and also does not change much over time. This indicates a longitudinal 'between-subjects' relationship between outcome variable Y and predictor variable X. Suppose that for another subject the value of the outcome variable Y increases rapidly along the longitudinal period, and suppose that for the same subject this pattern is also found for predictor variable X. This indicates a 'within-subject' relationship between outcome variable Y and predictor variable X. Both relationships

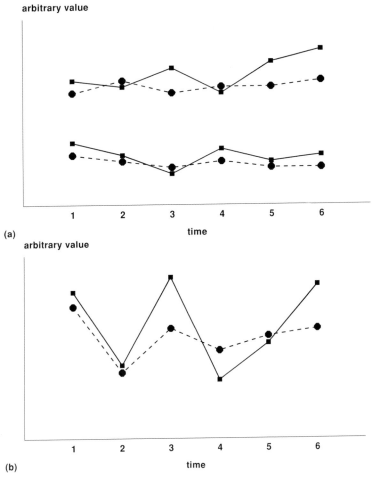

Figure 4.4. Illustration of the relationship between two continuous variables. The between-subjects relationship (a) and the within-subject relationship (b) (■ —— outcome variable, • – – – predictor variable).

are part of the overall longitudinal relationship between outcome variable Y and predictor variable X, so both should be taken into account in the analysis of the longitudinal relationship. The regression coefficient β_1 estimated with GEE analysis 'combines' the two possible relationships into one regression coefficient. Both phenomena are illustrated in Figure 4.4.

In Chapter 5, alternative models will be discussed with which it is possible to obtain an estimation of only the 'within-subject' relationships.

Table 4.1. Within-subject correlation structure for outcome variable Y

	Y_{t1}	Y_{t2}	Y_{t3}	Y_{t4}	Y_{t5}	Y_{t6}
Y_{t1}	—	0.76	0.70	0.67	0.64	0.59
Y_{t2}		—	0.77	0.78	0.67	0.59
Y_{t3}			—	0.85	0.71	0.63
Y_{t4}				—	0.74	0.65
Y_{t5}					—	0.69
Y_{t6}						—

4.5.4 Example

4.5.4.1 Introduction

Before carrying out a GEE analysis, the within-subject correlation structure must be chosen. As mentioned before, a possible choice for this working correlation structure can be based on the correlation structure of the observed data. Table 4.1 shows the observed correlation structure for outcome variable Y.

The first correlation structure that should be considered is an independent structure, i.e. all correlations are assumed to be zero. From Table 4.1 it can be seen that the lowest correlation coefficient is 0.59, i.e. far from zero, so an independent correlation structure does not appear to fit the observed data. The second possibility is an exchangeable structure, i.e. all correlations are assumed to be the same. The correlation coefficients range from 0.59 to 0.85. They are not equal, but they are generally of the same magnitude. Another possible correlation structure to consider is an m-dependent structure. With six repeated measurements, the highest order for an m-dependent structure is a 5-dependent structure (five time intervals). A lower-order-dependent structure does not appear to fit, because it implies that there are correlations close to zero, which is not the case in this particular situation. A 5-dependent correlation structure indicates that all correlations one measurement apart are equal, all correlations two measurements apart are equal, etc. Looking at the observed correlation structure, the correlations one measurement apart range from 0.69 to 0.85, the correlations two measurements apart range between 0.65 and 0.78, the correlations three measurements apart range between 0.63 and 0.67, and the correlations four measurements apart range between 0.59 and 0.64. In other words, a 5-dependent correlation structure fits the observed data quite well. From Table 4.1 it can be seen that an autoregressive correlation structure is less appropriate than a 5-dependent correlation structure. An autoregressive correlation structure assumes a steep decrease in correlation coefficients when the time interval between measurements increases. From Table 4.1 it can be seen that there is only a marginal decrease in the magnitude of the correlation coefficients with an increasing time interval. In every situation the unstructured correlation structure fits the data best, but it is questionable whether in this particular situation the loss of efficiency due to the estimation of 15 correlation coefficients is worthwhile – probably not.

So, neither an exchangeable structure nor a 5-dependent structure are perfect, but both seem to fit the observed data well. In such a situation, the working correlation structure for which the least number of parameters need to be estimated is the best choice. Therefore, in this particular situation an exchangeable structure is chosen.

Output 4.4. Results of a GEE analysis performed on the example dataset

```
Linear Generalized Estimating Equations
Response: YCONT   Corr: Exchangeable
Column Name        Coeff   StErr   p-value
--------------------------------------------
    0 Constant    3.617   0.680    0.000
    2 TIME        0.108   0.014    0.000
    4 X1         -0.024   0.274    0.931
    5 X2          0.111   0.023    0.000
    6 X3         -0.111   0.061    0.069
    7 X4          0.101   0.131    0.440
--------------------------------------------
n:147   s:0.747   #iter:12
Estimate of common correlation 0.562
```

4.5.4.2 Results of a GEE analysis

Output 4.4 shows the results of a GEE analysis that was applied to investigate the relationship between the outcome variable Y and the four predictor variables X_1 to X_4 and time. Time is added to the model as a continuous variable coded as [1, 2, 3, 4, 5, 6], assuming a linear relationship with time. This is (in principle) comparable to the within-subject time effect in MANOVA for repeated measurements, although the latter did not assume a linear relationship with time (see also Section 4.8).

The output is short, simple and straightforward. The first line of the output indicates that a linear GEE analysis was performed. The analysis is called 'linear', because a continuous outcome variable is analysed. In the second line, the outcome variable is mentioned (YCONT), together with the chosen correlation structure (exchangeable). The next part of the output contains the table with the regression coefficients, in which all the important information can be found. First of all, the column and name of the predictor variable are given. The column number refers to the column in which each specific variable was found in the dataset: the TIME variable was found in column 2 and the four predictor variables were found in columns 4 to 7. Although this is not important for the analysis, it shows directly that the data were organized in a 'long data structure' (see Section 1.6).

For each of the predictor variables the regression coefficient, the standard error of the coefficient and the corresponding p-value are given. The p-value is based on the Wald statistic, which is defined as the square of the ratio between the regression coefficient and its standard error. This statistic follows a χ^2 distribution with one degree of freedom, which is equal to the standard normal distribution squared. For example, for X_2 the Wald statistic is calculated as $(0.111/0.023)^2 = (4.83)^2$. According to the χ^2 distribution, the corresponding p-value is lower than 0.001. The interpretation of the magnitude of the regression coefficient is twofold: (1) the between-subjects interpretation indicates that a difference between two subjects of 1 unit in the predictor variable X_2 is associated with a difference of 0.111 units in the outcome variable Y; (2) the within-subject interpretation indicates that a change within one subject of 1 unit in the predictor variable X_2 is associated with a change of 0.111 units in the outcome variable Y. Again, the 'real' interpretation of the regression coefficient is a combination of both relationships. However, from the analysis that has been performed it is not possible to determine the contribution of each part.

From Output 4.4 it can be seen that X_2 is the only predictor variable which is significantly related to the development of outcome variable Y, and that this association is positive. For X_3 a negative association is found ($\beta = -0.111$), with a p-value close to the significance level of 5% ($p = 0.069$). The results also show that there is a significant linear increase over time of outcome variable Y ($\beta = 0.108$, $p < 0.001$), which was also concluded from the MANOVA for repeated measurements. So, again, in principle GEE analysis can provide the same information as MANOVA for repeated measurements with a 'one-within' design. Adding an interaction between X_4 and time to the GEE regression analysis will give similar information to MANOVA for repeated measurements with a 'one-within, one-between' design. It should be noted that in the simple GEE analysis a linear development over time is assumed. It is also possible to assume a quadratic development (or any other function) over time. To do so, a time squared (or any other function) term has to be added to the model analysed with GEE analysis. Another possibility is to treat the time variable as a categorical variable. The latter option will be discussed in Section 4.8.

In the last two lines of the output some additional information about the GEE model is given. The number of subjects ($n = 147$), the 'standard deviation of the model' ($s = 0.747$), which is also known as the scale parameter[2], and the number of iterations needed to obtain the estimates of the regression coefficients (#iter 12). With the 'variance of the model' an indication can be acquired for the 'explained variance' of the model. To obtain this indication, Equation (4.5) must be applied.

$$F_{it} = 1 - \left(\frac{S^2_{\text{model}}}{S^2_Y} \right) \tag{4.5}$$

where S^2_{model} is the variance of the model (given as s in the GEE output), and S^2_Y is the variance of the outcome variable Y, calculated over all available data.

The standard deviation of the outcome variable Y can be found in the descriptive information of the data, which is shown in Output 4.5. From Output 4.5 it can be seen that the standard deviation of outcome variable Y is 0.813. Applying Equation (4.5) to the data from the GEE analysis leads to an explained variance of $1 - (0.747)^2/(0.813)^2 = 15.6\%$. It should be stressed that this is only a vague indication of the explained variance of the model.

---

[2] The scale parameter is also known as the dispersion parameter, and is related to the way in which the variance of the outcome variable is related to the expected values of the outcome variable Y.

Output 4.5. Descriptive information of data used in the GEE analysis

DESC	($T)					
Col	Name	Size	Mean	StDev	Min	Max
1	ID	882	228.769	154.862	1.00	471.00
2	TIME	882	3.500	1.709	1.00	6.00
3	YCONT	882	4.500	0.813	2.40	7.50
4	X1	882	1.976	0.219	1.46	2.53
5	X2	882	3.743	1.530	1.57	12.21
6	X3	882	0.175	0.380	0.00	1.00
7	X4	882	1.531	0.499	1.00	2.00

The last line of the output of the GEE analysis gives an estimation of the common correlation, which is 0.562. This common correlation is an estimate of the correlation coefficient, which is used in the (exchangeable) working correlation structure. Although this value is used in the estimation of the regression coefficients, it is not important per se. From the output, the table of regression coefficients gives the really relevant information. In general, the regression coefficients, the standard errors (or a 95% confidence interval based on these standard errors ($\beta \pm 1.96$ times the standard error)) and the p-values are presented in the results of a GEE analysis.

4.5.4.3 Different correlation structures

Based on the observed correlation structure presented in Table 4.1, an exchangeable correlation structure was found to be the most appropriate choice in this particular situation. In Section 4.5 it was already mentioned that in the literature it is assumed that the GEE method is robust against a wrong choice of correlation structure. To verify this, the example dataset was reanalysed using different correlation structures. Output 4.6 shows the results of the GEE analysis with different correlation structures. The second lines of the outputs indicate the working correlation structures, and the estimated correlation coefficients are given in the last part of the outputs. For an independent correlation structure no correlation coefficients were estimated, while for a 5-dependent correlation structure five correlation coefficients were estimated. For the unstructured correlation structure, 15 different correlation coefficients were used in the analysis.

Output 4.6. Results of the GEE analysis with different correlation structures

```
Linear Generalized Estimating Equations
Response: YCONT  Corr: Independence
Column Name       Coeff StErr  p-value
----------------------------------------
    0 Constant   3.247 0.672    0.000
    2 TIME       0.089 0.014    0.000
    4 X1         0.113 0.270    0.675
    5 X2         0.173 0.026    0.000
    6 X3        -0.016 0.093    0.860
    7 X4         0.046 0.131    0.728
----------------------------------------
n:147  s:0.742   #iter:12

Linear Generalized Estimating Equations
Response: YCONT   Corr: 5-Dependence
Column Name       Coeff StErr  p-value
----------------------------------------
    0 Constant   3.667 0.689    0.000
    2 TIME       0.127 0.014    0.000
    4 X1        -0.074 0.277    0.790
    5 X2         0.087 0.023    0.000
    6 X3        -0.104 0.061    0.091
    7 X4         0.132 0.132    0.315
----------------------------------------
n:147  s:0.752   #iter:16
Estimate of common correlations 0.667, 0.524, 0.485, 0.582, 0.79

Linear Generalized Estimating Equations
Response: YCONT Corr: Unspecified
Column Name       Coeff StErr  p-value
----------------------------------------
    0 Constant   3.780 0.714    0.000
    2 TIME       0.089 0.013    0.000
    4 X1        -0.009 0.289    0.976
    5 X2         0.106 0.023    0.000
    6 X3        -0.094 0.057    0.096
    7 X4         0.092 0.136    0.496
----------------------------------------
n:147  s:0.755   #iter:13
Estimate of common correlation
1.000   0.758   0.692   0.652   0.600   0.552
0.758   1.000   0.759   0.761   0.628   0.566
0.692   0.759   1.000   0.821   0.673   0.620
0.652   0.761   0.821   1.000   0.692   0.617
0.600   0.628   0.673   0.692   1.000   0.648
0.552   0.566   0.620   0.617   0.648   1.000
```

Table 4.2. Regression coefficients and standard errors estimated by GEE analysis with different correlation structures

		Correlation structure		
	Independent	5-Dependent	Exchangeable	Unstructured
X_1	0.11 (0.27)	−0.07 (0.27)	−0.02 (0.27)	−0.01 (0.29)
X_2	0.17 (0.03)	0.09 (0.02)	0.11 (0.02)	0.11 (0.02)
X_3	−0.02 (0.09)	−0.11 (0.06)	−0.11 (0.06)	−0.09 (0.06)
X_4	0.05 (0.13)	0.13 (0.13)	0.10 (0.13)	0.09 (0.14)
Time	0.09 (0.01)	0.13 (0.01)	0.11 (0.01)	0.09 (0.01)

Table 4.2 summarizes the results of the analysis with different working correlation structures. From Table 4.2 it can be seen that, although the conclusions based on p-values are the same, there are some differences in the magnitude of the regression coefficients. This is important, because it is far more interesting to estimate the magnitude of the association by means of the regression coefficients and the 95% confidence intervals than just estimating p-values. Based on the results of Table 4.2, it is obvious that it is important to choose a suitable correlation structure before a GEE analysis is performed.

To put the importance of correcting for the dependency of observations in a broader perspective the results of the GEE analysis can be compared to a 'naive' longitudinal analysis, ignoring the fact that repeated observations are carried out on the same subjects (i.e. a linear regression analysis carried out on a total longitudinal dataset). Output 4.7 shows the results of such a 'naive' linear regression analysis carried out on the example dataset.

A comparison between Output 4.6 (Table 4.2) and Output 4.7 indicates that the regression coefficients obtained from the 'naive' longitudinal analysis are exactly the same as the regression coefficients obtained from a GEE analysis with an independent correlation structure. The standard errors of the regression coefficients are however totally different. In general, ignoring the dependency of the observations leads to an under-estimation of the standard errors of the time-independent predictor variables and an over-estimation of the standard errors of the time-dependent predictor variables. For the time-independent predictor variables in the naive analysis, it is assumed that each measurement within a particular subject provides 100% new information, while part of the information was already available in

Output 4.7. Results of a 'naive' linear regression analysis performed on the example dataset

```
Linear Regression Analysis
Response: YCONT
Column    Name          Coeff    StErr    p-value           SS
-------------------------------------------------------------------
    0     Constant      3.247    0.357     0.000     17858.699
    2     TIME          0.089    0.016     0.000        41.034
    4     X1            0.113    0.145     0.433         8.968
    5     X2            0.173    0.020     0.000        49.288
    6     X3           -0.016    0.069     0.814         0.051
    7     X4            0.046    0.064     0.479         0.277
-------------------------------------------------------------------
df:876    RSq:0.171     s:0.742      RSS:482.461
```

earlier measurements of that subject, reflected in the within-subject cor-relation coefficient. Depending on the magnitude of that coefficient, each repeated measurement within one subject provides less than 100% new information. This leads to larger standard errors in the corrected analysis. For the time-dependent predictor variables, however, GEE analysis makes use of the fact that the same subjects are measured over time. This leads to lower standard errors of the regression coefficients.

4.5.4.4 Unequally spaced time intervals

Because time is one of the predictor variables in the model used to analyse the relationships between outcome variable Y and several predictor variables (Equation (4.3)), it is simple to add unequally spaced time intervals to the model. Suppose that in the example dataset, the first four measurements were carried out at yearly intervals, and the fifth and sixth measurements at 5-year intervals. So, time must be coded as [1, 2, 3, 4, 9, 14] instead of [1, 2, 3, 4, 5, 6]. When such a dataset is considered, the results of the GEE analysis change considerably (see Output 4.8).

It is expected that the relationship between the outcome variable Y and time changes when the time intervals are unequally spaced. It is import-ant to realize that the relationship with the other four predictor variables also changes (see Figure 4.5). For predictor variable X_3 (a dichotomous

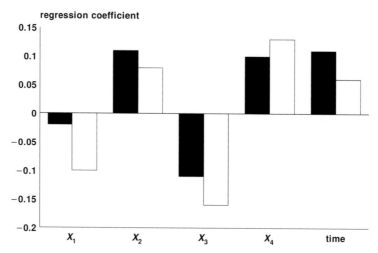

Figure 4.5. Regression coefficients estimated by GEE analysis with a dataset with equally spaced time intervals (■) and a dataset with unequally spaced time intervals (□).

Output 4.8. Results of the GEE analysis with a dataset with unequally spaced time intervals

```
Linear Generalized Estimating Equations
Response: YCONT  Corr: Exchangeable
Column  Name         Coeff   StErr   p-value
-------------------------------------------
     0  Constant     3.900   0.693    0.000
     2  TIME         0.060   0.005    0.000
     4  X1          -0.098   0.279    0.727
     5  X2           0.077   0.020    0.000
     6  X3          -0.161   0.054    0.003
     7  X4           0.131   0.132    0.322
-------------------------------------------
n:147  s:0.731  #iter:12
Estimate of common correlation 0.621
```

time-dependent predictor variable), for instance, when the repeated measurements were equally spaced a non-significant result was found, while when the repeated measurements were unequally spaced a highly significant relationship was observed. These differences emphasize the importance of adding an actual time indicator to the statistical model, especially when the time intervals are unequally spaced (see also Section 4.8).

4.6 Random coefficient analysis

4.6.1 Introduction

Random coefficient analysis is also known as multilevel analysis or mixed-effect analysis (Laird and Ware, 1982; Longford, 1993; Goldstein, 1995). Multilevel analysis was initially developed in the social sciences, more specifically for educational research. Investigating the performance of pupils in schools, researchers realized that the performances of pupils within the same class are not independent, i.e. their performances are more or less correlated. Similarly, the performances of classes within the same school can be dependent on each other. This type of study design is characterized by a hierarchical structure. Students are nested within classes, and classes are nested within schools. Various levels can be distinguished. Because the performances of pupils within one class are not independent of each other, a correction should be made for this dependency in the analysis of the performance of the pupils. Multilevel analysis is developed to correct for this dependency, for instance by allowing for different regression coefficients for different classes. As this technique is suitable for correlated observations, it is obvious that it is also suitable for use in longitudinal studies. In longitudinal studies the observations within one subject over time are correlated. The observations over time are nested within the subject. The basic idea behind the use of multilevel techniques in longitudinal studies is that the regression coefficients are allowed to differ between subjects. Therefore the term random coefficient analysis is preferred to the term multilevel analysis.

4.6.2 Random coefficient analysis in longitudinal studies

The simplest form of random coefficient analysis is an analysis with only a random intercept. The corresponding statistical model with which to analyse a longitudinal relationship between an outcome variable Y and time is given in Equation (4.6).

$$Y_{it} = \beta_{0i} + \beta_1 t + \varepsilon_{it} \tag{4.6}$$

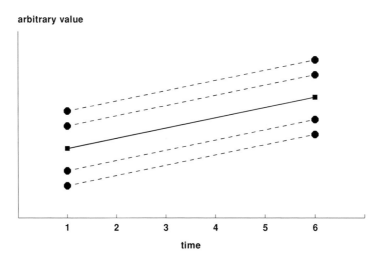

arbitrary value

time

Figure 4.6. Development over time of a particular outcome variable Y; different intercepts for different subjects ($\blacksquare$ —— population, $\bullet$ – – – individuals 1 to n).

where Y_{it} are observations for subject i at time t, β_{0i} is the random intercept, t is time, β_1 is the regression coefficient for time, and ε_{it} is the 'error' for subject i at time t. What is new about this model (compared to Equation (4.2)) is the random intercept β_{0i}, i.e. the intercept can vary between subjects. Figure 4.6 illustrates this phenomenon.

It is also possible that the intercept is not random, but that the development of a certain variable over time is allowed to vary among subjects or, in other words, the 'slope' with time is considered to be random. This phenomenon is illustrated in Figure 4.7 and in Equation (4.7).

$$Y_{it} = \beta_0 + \beta_{1i}t + \varepsilon_{it} \tag{4.7}$$

where Y_{it} are observations for subject i at time t, β_0 is the intercept, t is time, β_{1i} is the random regression coefficient for time, and ε_{it} is the 'error' for subject i at time t.

The most interesting possibility is the combination of a random intercept and a random slope with time, which is illustrated in Figure 4.8 and Equation (4.8).

$$Y_{it} = \beta_{0i} + \beta_{1i}t + \varepsilon_{it} \tag{4.8}$$

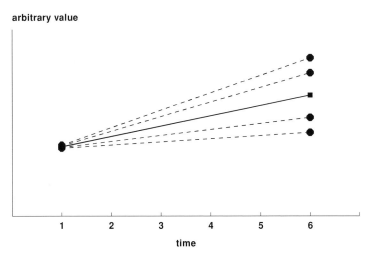

Figure 4.7. Development over time of a particular outcome variable Y; different slopes for different subjects (■ —— population, • – – – individuals 1 to n).

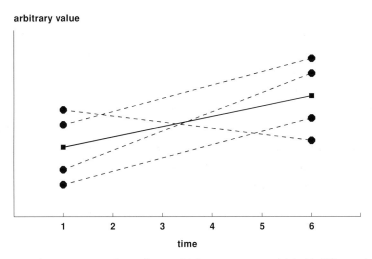

Figure 4.8. Development over time of a particular outcome variable Y; different intercepts and different slopes for different subjects (■ —— population, • – – – individuals 1 to n).

where Y_{it} are observations for subject i at time t, β_{0i} is the random intercept, t is time, β_{1i} is the random regression coefficient for time, and ε_{it} is the 'error' for subject i at time t.

Up to now, random coefficient models have been discussed in the light of the description of the development of a certain outcome variable Y over time.

In fact, these models can be extended to form random regression models in order to describe the longitudinal relationship between a continuous outcome variable and several other variables (Equation (4.9)).

$$Y_{it} = \beta_{0i} + \sum_{j=1}^{J} \beta_{1ij} X_{itj} + \beta_{2i} t + \sum_{k=1}^{K} \beta_{3ik} Z_{ikt} + \sum_{m=1}^{M} \beta_{4im} G_{im} + \varepsilon_{it} \qquad (4.9)$$

where Y_{it} are observations for subject i at time t, β_{0i} is the random intercept, X_{ijt} is the independent variable j for subject i at time t, β_{1ij} is the random regression coefficient for independent variable j, J is the number of independent variables, t is time, β_{2i} is the random regression coefficient for time, Z_{ikt} is the time-dependent covariate k for subject i at time t, β_{3ik} is the random regression coefficient for time-dependent covariate k, K is the number of time-dependent covariates, G_{im} is the time-independent covariate m for subject i, β_{4im} is the random regression coefficient for time-independent covariate m, M is the number of time-independent covariates, and ε_{it} is the 'error' for subject i at time t.

The model used in Equation (4.9) is almost identical to the model used in Equation (4.3), the difference being that in the model used for random coefficient analysis, the regression coefficients are allowed to vary between subjects, and in Equation (4.3) this was not the case. The assumption of random coefficient analysis is that the variation in intercept and variation in slopes are normally distributed with an average of zero and a certain variance. This variance is estimated by the statistical software package.

The general idea of random coefficient analysis is that the unexplained variance in outcome variable Y is divided into different components. One of the components is related to the random intercept and another component is related to random slopes (Figure (4.9)).

4.6.3 Example

4.6.3.1 Results of a random coefficient analysis

Output 4.9 shows the results of the analysis in which the outcome variable Y is only related to time and in which a random intercept is modelled (Equation (4.6)). The first part of the output gives an overview of the dataset (e.g. number of observations, number of subjects) and the analysis performed. The first line refers to the fact that a random effects ML regression

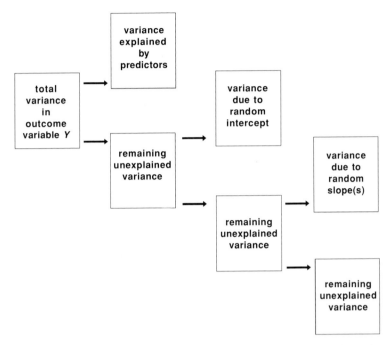

Figure 4.9. Schematic illustration of random coefficient analysis; the unexplained variance in outcome variable *Y* is divided into different components.

Output 4.9. Results of random coefficient analysis with a random intercept

```
Random-effects ML regression              Number of obs      =      882
Group variable (i) : id                   Number of groups   =      147
Random effects u_i ~ Gaussian             Obs per group: min =        6
                                                         avg =      6.0
                                                         max =        6
                                          LR chi2(1)         =   149.34
Log likelihood = -804.40727               Prob > chi2        =   0.0000
-----------------------------------------------------------------------
   ycont      Coeff   Std. Err.      z    P > |z|   [95% Conf.  Interval]
-----------------------------------------------------------------------
    time   0.1262974  0.0098144  12.869   0.000    0.1070615  0.1455333
   _cons   4.057732   0.0628345  64.578   0.000    3.934579   4.180886
-----------------------------------------------------------------------
/sigma_u   0.6046707  0.0392889  15.390   0.000    0.5276658  0.6816757
/sigma_e   0.4977992  0.0129827  38.343   0.000    0.4723536  0.5232448
-----------------------------------------------------------------------
     rho   0.5960358  0.0342401                    0.5278381  0.6614276
-----------------------------------------------------------------------
Likelihood ratio test of sigma_u=0: chi2(1) = 463.17  Prob > chi2 = 0.0000
```

has been performed. The ML stands for maximum likelihood, which is the estimation procedure used in this example. Furthermore, from the first part of the output it can be seen that the random regression coefficient (i.e. intercept) is normally distributed (random effects u_i $\sim$ Gaussian). It also gives the log likelihood value of the model and a likelihood ratio test (LR chi2(1)) and the corresponding p-value (Prob > chi2). The log likelihood is an indication of the adequacy (or 'fit') of the model. The value by itself is useless, but can be used in the likelihood ratio test. The interpretations of the log likelihood and the likelihood ratio test are exactly the same as known from logistic regression analysis (Hosmer and Lemeshow, 1989; Kleinbaum, 1994). The likelihood ratio test shown in this part of the output is a test to evaluate the significance of the regression coefficients. In other words, it is a test to evaluate the importance of the time variable in the model. In principle, this test is based on the difference in -2 log likelihood between the model presented and the model without time, i.e. with only an intercept. Presumably this difference in -2 log likelihood is 149.34. This difference follows a χ^2 distribution with one degree of freedom, which gives a value $p < 0.001$.

The second part of the output shows the regression coefficients. In this simple example, only the relationship with time was analysed, so only the regression coefficients for time and the intercept are given. The information provided is comparable to the information obtained from a normal linear regression analysis and the earlier discussed GEE analysis: the regression coefficient (0.1262974), the corresponding standard error (0.0098144), the z-statistic (calculated as the regression coefficient divided by the standard error, i.e. 12.869), the p-value belonging to the z-statistic (0.000) and the 95% confidence interval around the regression coefficient (0.1070615 to 0.1455333). The latter is calculated in the usual way (i.e. the regression coefficient ± 1.96 times the standard error).

Below the regression coefficients the values of /sigma_u and /sigma_e are presented. This part provides information about the random part of the model. In general, the idea of random coefficient analysis is that the overall 'error' variance is divided into different parts (see Figure 4.9). In this simple example, the overall 'error' variance is divided into two parts, one which is related to the random variation in the intercept (i.e. /sigma_u), and one which is the remaining 'error' variance (i.e. /sigma_e). The STATA output does not give the variances, but the standard deviations (indicated by /sigma). The variances can easily be obtained by calculating the square of the standard deviations. The last coefficient shown is rho, which is an estimation of the intraclass correlation coefficient (ICC). The ICC is calculated as the variance of the intercepts (i.e. (sigma_u)^2) divided by the total variance (which is the sum of (sigma_u)^2 and (sigma_e)^2). The ICC can be used as an indication of the within-subject dependency.

The last line of the output gives the results of another likelihood ratio test. This likelihood ratio test is related to the random part of the model, and for this test, the -2 log likelihood of the presented model is compared to the -2 log likelihood which would have been found if the same analysis was performed without a random intercept. Apparently, the difference in -2 log likelihood between the two models is 463.17, which follows a χ^2 distribution with one degree of freedom; one degree of freedom, because the difference in parameters between the two models compared is one (i.e. the random variation in intercepts sigma_u). This value is highly significant (Prob > chi2 = 0.0000), which indicates that in this situation a random intercept should be considered. In the coefficient table in which the two variance components were given, for each standard deviation the standard error, the z-statistic, the corresponding p-value and the 95% confidence interval were also shown. It is very tempting to use the z-statistic of the random variation in intercepts to evaluate the importance of considering a random intercept. However, one must realize that the z-statistic is a normal approximation, which is not very valid, especially in the evaluation of variance parameters. In other words, it is advised to use the likelihood ratio test to evaluate the importance of allowing random coefficients.

To verify the importance of a random intercept, Output 4.10 shows the results of an analysis in which no random coefficient is considered. First of all, it can be seen that the total error variance (i.e. dispersion 0.6148249) is the sum of the two error variances shown in Output 4.9. Secondly, the log likelihood of this model is -1035.99227, which produces a -2 log likelihood of 2071.98. Performing the likelihood ratio test between the model with and without a random intercept gives (as expected from Output (4.9)) a value of 463.17, which is highly significant.

Output 4.10. Results of a 'naive' regression analysis with no random intercept

```
Log likelihood = -1035.99227
Residual df     =         880        No. of obs =         882
Pearson X2      =    541.0459        Deviance   =   541.0459
Dispersion      =   0.6148249        Dispersion =  0.6148249
Gaussian (normal) distribution, identity link
-----------------------------------------------------------------
ycont      Coeff Std. Err.    t    P > |t| [95% Conf.  Interval]
-----------------------------------------------------------------
 time  0.1262974  0.0154596   8.170  0.000   0.0959554   0.1566394
_cons  4.057732   0.0602065  67.397  0.000   3.939567    4.175897
```

In the two models considered, the β_1 coefficient describing the relationship between outcome variable Y and time is considered to be fixed (i.e. not assumed to vary between subjects). The next step in the modelling process is to add a random slope to the model, i.e. to let β_1 vary among subjects (Equation (4.7)). The result of a random coefficient analysis with such a model is shown in Output 4.11.

Output 4.11. Results of random coefficient analyses with a random intercept and a random slope

```
log likelihood = -795.25898
-----------------------------------------------------------------
ycont      Coeff Std. Err.    z    P > |z| [95% Conf. Interval]
-----------------------------------------------------------------
time   0.1263673  0.0111119  11.372  0.000   0.1045884   0.1481463
_cons  4.060211   0.0560216  72.476  0.000   3.95041     4.170011
-----------------------------------------------------------------
Variance at level 1
-----------------------------------------------------------------
0.23010497 (0.01355609)

Variances and covariances of random effects
-----------------------------------------------------------------
***level 2 (id)
  var(1): 0.262258 (0.05560083)
cov(1,2): 0.00610365 (0.00892569)  cor(1,2): 0.16848744
  var(2): 0.00500397 (0.00239667)
```

This output looks slightly different to the output shown earlier for the situation with a random intercept. It is less extensive, but the important information is provided. First of all, the log likelihood is given (i.e. -795.25898). This is the likelihood value related to the total model, including both regression coefficients and variance components. This value can be used to evaluate the importance of the inclusion of a random slope in the model. Therefore, the -2 log likelihood of this model must be compared to the -2 log likelihood of the model without a random slope. The difference between the -2 log likelihoods is $1608.8 - 1590.5 = 18.3$. This value follows a χ^2-distribution with a number of degrees of freedom equal to the difference in the number of parameters estimated by the two models. Although only a random slope is added to the model, **two** extra parameters are estimated. Obviously, one of the estimated parameters is the variance of the slopes, and the other (not so obviously) is the covariance between the random intercept and the random slope. This can be seen from the last part of the output. First of all, the variance at level 1 is given. This is the remaining overall error variance (i.e. $(\text{sigma\_e})^2$). Secondly, the variances and covariances of random effects are given. The first variance given ($\text{var}(1)$ 0.262258 (0.05560083)) is an estimation of the random variation in intercepts with the corresponding standard error, while the second variance ($\text{var}(2)$ 0.00500397 (0.00239667)) provides the same information for the random variation in slopes. The output also gives the $\text{cov}(1,2)$ (0.00610365 (0.00892569)) and the $\text{cor}(1,2)$ (0.16848744). These are values indicating the covariance and correlation between the random intercept and random slope. The magnitude and direction of the covariance/correlation between random intercept and random slope give information about the interaction between random intercept and slope. When a negative correlation is found, subjects with a high intercept have lower slopes. When a positive correlation is found, subjects with a high intercept also have a high slope (see Figure 4.10).

Because the correlation is calculated from the covariance, the model with a random slope has two more parameters than the model with only a random intercept. So, the value calculated earlier with the likelihood ratio test (i.e. 18.3) follows a χ^2 distribution with two degrees of freedom. This value is highly significant, so in this situation not only a random intercept seems to be important, but also a random slope.

The next step is to add the predictor variables to the statistical model, in order to investigate the relationship between outcome variable Y and the four

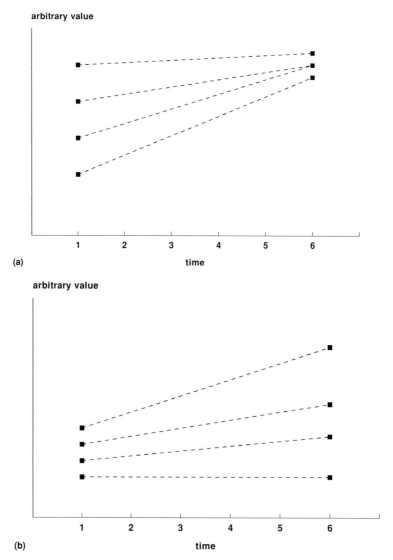

Figure 4.10. (a) Negative correlation between slope and intercept, (b) positive correlation between slope and intercept.

predictor variables X_1 to X_4. Output 4.12 shows the results of the random coefficient analysis.

From Output 4.12 it can be seen that the four predictor variables X_1 to X_4 are assumed to be fixed. There are no more random variances estimated than in the analysis shown in Output 4.11. This is not really necessary but

Output 4.12. Results of random coefficient analyses with a random intercept and a random slope with time in order to investigate the relationship between outcome variable Y and the four predictor variables X_1 to X_4

```
log likelihood = -778.89879
------------------------------------------------------------------------
  ycont        Coeff    Std. Err.     z     P > |z|   [95% Conf.   Interval]
------------------------------------------------------------------------
   time      0.1098585   0.0122515    8.967   0.000    0.085846    0.1338711
     x1     -0.0244138   0.2705055   -0.090   0.928   -0.5545948   0.5057672
     x2      0.1070983   0.0206451    5.188   0.000    0.0666346   0.147562
     x3     -0.1206264   0.0597928   -2.017   0.044   -0.2378181  -0.0034346
     x4      0.0415465   0.1202568    0.345   0.730   -0.1941526   0.2772455
   _cons     3.721137    0.6609747    5.630   0.000    2.425651    5.016624
------------------------------------------------------------------------

Variance at level 1
------------------------------------------------------------------------
0.22480938 (0.01311782)

Variances and covariances of random effects
------------------------------------------------------------------------
***level 2 (id)
  var(1):   0.26543988 (0.05671975)
cov(1,2): -0.00049603 (0.00908093) cor(1,2): -0.01395848
  var(2):   0.00475738 (0.00217723)
```

seems to be appropriate in most situations. Because all regression coefficients related to the predictor variables are assumed to be fixed, the output from the last analysis looks similar to that in Output 4.11. The difference is that now the relationships between outcome variable Y and the four predictor variables are estimated. The coefficients can be tested for significance with the z-statistic, which has been described earlier. For instance, for X_2 the regression coefficient (0.107) divided by the standard error (0.021) gives a z-statistic of 5.188, which is highly significant. For the other variables the same procedure can be followed. The log likelihood value obtained by this analysis is (again) the likelihood of the total model. A comparison between the -2 log likelihood of this model and the -2 log likelihood derived from the analysis presented in Output 4.11 gives an indication of the importance of **all** predictor variables. In this example, the difference between the -2 log likelihoods is 32.72, which follows a χ^2 distribution with four degrees of freedom (four predictor variables were added and no extra random regression coefficients).

This likelihood ratio test gives $p < 0.001$. It should be noted that the likelihood values of two different models can only be compared with each other when one model is an extension of the other model.

The interpretation of the regression coefficients of the four predictor variables from a random coefficient analysis is exactly the same as the interpretation of the regression coefficients estimated with GEE analysis, so the interpretation is twofold: (1) the 'between-subjects' interpretation indicates that a difference between two subjects of 1 unit in, for instance, the predictor variable X_2 is associated with a difference of 0.107 units in the outcome variable Y; (2) the 'within-subject' interpretation indicates that a change within one subject of 1 unit in the predictor variable X_2 is associated with a change of 0.107 units in the outcome variable Y. Again, the 'real' interpretation is a combination of both relationships.

The way the analysis is built up in this example, it is possible that owing to some of the predictor variables added to the model, the variance due to the random intercept and/or random slopes is no longer important. So, in fact, the necessity of a random intercept and random slope(s) should be re-investigated with the total model, i.e. the model with the four predictor variables. Therefore, firstly the results of the analysis given in Output 4.12 can be compared with the results obtained from an analysis with the four predictor variables but without a random slope with time. Secondly, the results can be compared with the results obtained from an analysis with the four predictor variables but without a random intercept.

4.6.3.2 Unequally spaced time intervals

What has been seen in the results of the GEE analysis performed on a dataset with unequally spaced time intervals is exactly the same for the results of the random coefficient analysis (Figure 4.11). There are striking differences between the results of the dataset with equally spaced time intervals and the results of the dataset with unequally spaced time intervals. Not only has the regression coefficient of time changed considerably, but the regression coefficients of the four predictor variables have also changed.

4.6.4 Comments

In the first lines of the outputs it was indicated that a maximum likelihood estimation procedure had been performed. There is some debate in

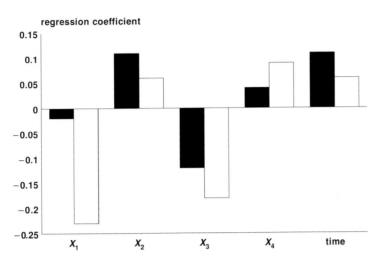

Figure 4.11. Regression coefficients estimated by random coefficient analysis with a dataset with equally spaced time intervals (■) and a dataset with unequally spaced time intervals (□).

the literature about whether maximum likelihood is the best way to estimate the regression coefficients in a random coefficient analysis. Some statisticians believe that restricted maximum likelihood is a better estimation procedure. It is also argued that maximum likelihood estimation is more suitable for the estimation of the fixed effects (i.e. for estimation of the regression coefficients), while restricted maximum likelihood estimation is more suitable for estimation of the different variance components (Harville, 1977; Laird and Ware, 1982; Pinheiro and Bates, 2000). It should be realized that in practice one is interested more in the regression coefficients than in the magnitude of the variance components.

To facilitate the discussion, all the models have been restricted to simple linear models, i.e. no squared terms, no complicated relationships with time, no difficult interactions, etc. This does not mean that it is not possible to use more complicated models. When looking at possible interaction terms, special attention must be paid to the interactions between each of the predictor variables with time. These interactions indicate in which part of the longitudinal period the observed relationships are the strongest. To illustrate the interpretation of an interaction with time, an interaction between X_2 and time was added to the model described in Output 4.12. Output 4.13 shows the results of the analysis.

Output 4.13. Results of a random coefficient analysis, with an interaction between X_2 and time

```
log likelihood = -757.23705
```

ycont	Coeff	Std. Err.	z	P > |z|	[95% Conf.	Interval]
x1	-0.2433723	0.2870338	-0.848	0.397	-0.8059483	0.3192036
x2	-0.1022496	0.0374449	-2.731	0.006	-0.1756403	-0.0288589
x3	-0.1185118	0.0579058	-2.047	0.041	-0.2320051	-0.0050186
x4	0.0790463	0.1224855	0.645	0.519	-0.1610209	0.3191136
time	-0.0670296	0.0293231	-2.286	0.022	-0.1245018	-0.0095573
inttx2	0.0493359	0.0074909	6.586	0.000	0.0346539	0.0640179
_cons	4.821793	0.7090097	6.801	0.000	3.43216	6.211427

```
Variance at level 1
------------------------------------------------------------------
0.21329023 (.01271139)

Variances and covariances of random effects
------------------------------------------------------------------
***level 2 (id)
  var(1):   0.2979293 (0.06051497)
cov(1,2): -0.0005461 (0.00943201)  cor(1,2): -0.0178419
  var(2):   0.00314448 (0.00219192)
```

The most interesting part of the output is the importance of the interaction between X_2 and time. This can be evaluated in two ways: firstly with the z-statistic of the interaction term, and secondly with the likelihood ratio test between the model with the interaction and the model without the interaction. The z-statistic for the interaction term has a value of 6.586, and a corresponding p-value of 0.000, i.e. highly significant. The likelihood ratio test is based on the difference between the -2 log likelihood of the model without an interaction (from Output 4.12 the -2 log likelihood can be calculated as 1557.8) and the -2 log likelihood of the model with an interaction (from Output 4.13 the -2 log likelihood can be calculated as 1514.4). This difference is 43.4, which follows a χ^2 distribution with one (i.e. the interaction term) degree of freedom, which is highly significant. In general, for evaluation of the regression coefficients, the z-statistic produces similar results to the likelihood ratio test, but the latter is assumed to be slightly better. The significant interaction between X_2 and time indicates that the relationship between X_2 and the outcome variable Y differs along the longitudinal period. The sign of the regression coefficient related to the interaction term is positive. This suggests that the relationship between X_2 and Y becomes stronger as time increases. In fact, from Output 4.13, the magnitude of the relationship between X_2 and Y at each of the different time-points can be estimated by combining the regression coefficient for X_2 and the regression coefficient for the interaction term.

4.7 Comparison between GEE analysis and random coefficient analysis

In the foregoing paragraphs the general ideas behind GEE analysis and random coefficient analysis were discussed. Both methods are highly suitable for the analysis of longitudinal data, because in both methods a correction is made for the dependency of the observations within one subject: in GEE analysis by assuming a certain working correlation structure, and in random coefficient analysis by allowing the regression coefficients to vary between subjects. The question then arises: Which of the two methods is better? Which method is the most appropriate to answer the research question: 'What is the relationship between the development of outcome variable Y and several predictor variables X?' Unfortunately, no clear answer can be given. In principle, GEE analysis with an exchangeable correlation structure is the same as random coefficient analysis with only a random intercept. The correction for the dependency of observations with an exchangeable 'working correlation' structure is the same as allowing subjects to have random intercepts. When an exchangeable correlation structure is not appropriate, GEE analysis with a different correlation structure can be used. When an exchangeable correlation structure is appropriate, and there is no random variation in one of the estimated regression coefficients (except the intercept), GEE analysis and random coefficient analysis are equally appropriate. When there is significant and relevant random variation in one (or more) of the regression coefficients, random coefficient analysis can be used, with the additional possibility of allowing other coefficients to vary between subjects.

It is very important to realize that the differences and equalities between GEE analysis and random coefficient analysis described in this section only hold for continuous outcome variables. For dichotomous and categorical outcome variables, the situation is different (see Chapters 6 and 7).

4.7.1 Extensions of random coefficient analysis

To summarize, a GEE analysis with an exchangeable correlation structure is the same as a random coefficient analysis with only a random intercept. The assumption of random coefficient analysis is that the random intercepts between individuals are normally distributed with mean zero and a certain variance (which is estimated by the statistical software package and given in the output). Although this assumption is quite sufficient in many situations, sometimes the random variation is not normally distributed. Therefore, some software packages (e.g. STATA) provide the possibility of modelling (to some extent) the distribution of the variation in the regression coefficients (see for instance Rabe-Hesketh et al., 2001a).

In GEE analysis there is some flexibility in modelling the correlation structure, which is not available in 'standard' random coefficient analysis. Therefore, in some software packages (e.g. S-PLUS), the random coefficient analysis can be extended by adding a correlation structure to the model. The possible correlation structures are basically the same as has been described for GEE analysis (see Section 4.5.2). In fact, this additional correction can be carried out when the random coefficients are not sufficient to correct for the dependency of observations. In more technical terms, despite the correction made by the random coefficients, the 'error' is still correlated within subjects, which indicates that an additional correction is necessary.

Although this additional correction is an interesting extension of the 'standard' random coefficient analysis, it should be used with caution. This is mostly because there is a danger of 'over-correction'. It is for instance possible to model both a random intercept and an additional exchangeable correlation structure. Because the two options are exactly the same, this will lead to 'over-correction' and corresponding problems with the estimation and interpretation of the regression coefficients.

4.7.2 Equal variances over time

With GEE analysis only one variance parameter is estimated. This suggests more or less that the variance in outcome variable Y remains equal over time. This is, however, not always true. It is very likely that in a longitudinal study a change in variance over time in the outcome variable Y occurs. This phenomenon is also known as 'heteroscedasticity'. In random coefficient analysis the change in variance over time in the outcome variable Y is (partly) taken into account by the possibility of a random slope. It is, however, possible that a random slope is not sufficient to correct for the changing variance over time. Or in other words, despite the correction due to the random slope, the 'error variance' is still changing over time. Therefore, in some software packages (e.g. S-PLUS) additional modelling of the variance over time is possible. This is done by adding a certain 'variance function' to the random coefficient model. For more information reference should be made to for instance Pinheiro and Bates (2000).

4.7.2.1 A numerical example

It is interesting to illustrate the influence of a changing variance over time on the magnitude of the regression coefficients of a simple longitudinal data analysis. Consider the two (simple) longitudinal datasets shown in Figure 4.12. In both datasets nine subjects were measured twice in time.

In the first longitudinal dataset, there is an increase of the variance in outcome variable YVAR1 at the follow-up measurement, while in the second longitudinal dataset (YVAR2), there is a decrease in variance over time. For both datasets the research question is related to the development over time. Both datasets are analysed with GEE analysis, with random coefficient analysis with only a random intercept, and with random coefficient analysis with a random intercept and a random slope. Table 4.3 shows the results of the analyses.

It is not surprising that the results of the GEE analysis and the random coefficient analysis with only a random intercept are exactly the same. Furthermore, it is also not surprising that the regression coefficients for time are more or less the same for all three analyses. The difference between GEE analysis and random coefficient analysis with both a random intercept and a random slope is observed in the standard error of the regression coefficient for time. Allowing a random slope leads to a decrease in the standard error of the regression coefficient. In other words, it leads to a more efficient estimate of the standard error.

4.7.3 The correction for covariance

In some software packages (e.g. SAS) the correction for the correlated observations and the (possible) changing variance over time is combined in a correction for the 'covariance'. The 'covariance' between two measurements

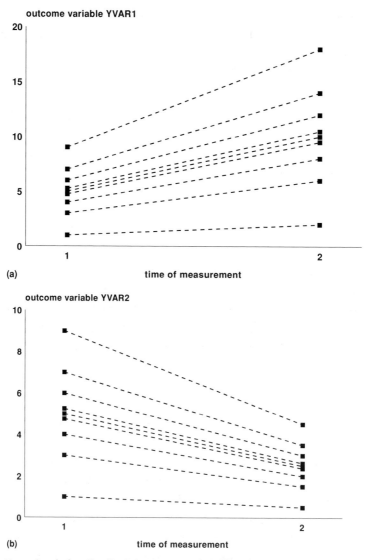

Figure 4.12. Two simple longitudinal datasets used to illustrate the influence of a changing variance over time; one dataset with an increase in variance over time (a) and one dataset with a decrease in variance over time (b).

is a combination of the correlation between the two measurements and the variances of the two measurements (Equation 4.10).

$$\text{covar}\,(Y_t,\,Y_{t+1}) = \text{corr}\,(Y_t,\,Y_{t+1})\,\text{sd}\,(Y_t)\,\text{sd}\,(Y_{t+1})\qquad\qquad(4.10)$$

Table 4.3. Regression coefficients and standard errors (in parentheses) for time estimated with different analyses on two (simple) longitudinal datasets given in Figure 4.12

	GEE analysis	Random coefficient analysis with random intercept	Random coefficient analysis with random intercept and slope
YVAR1	5.00 (0.63)	5.00 (0.63)	5.02 (0.43)
YVAR2	−2.50 (0.31)	−2.50 (0.31)	−2.50 (0.24)

where $\text{covar}(Y_t, Y_{t+1})$ is the covariance between Y at t and Y at $t+1$, $\text{corr}(Y_t, Y_{t+1})$ is the correlation between Y at t and Y at $t+1$, and $\text{sd}(Y_t)$ is the standard deviation of Y at t.

Comparable to the correction for the correlation between the observations used in GEE, there are many different possibilities for the correction for the 'covariance' between observations (see Chapter 12 for details). Again, basically the correction is made for the 'error covariance', which is equal to the covariance of the repeated observations in an analysis without any predictor variables.

4.7.4 Comments

In the foregoing sections it was often mentioned that sophisticated analyses are needed to correct for correlated observations. However, basically the correction in longitudinal data analysis is carried out for correlated 'errors'. The same holds for the changing variance over time. When there are no predictor variables in the model, the correlation and changing variance over time are equivalent to the same phenomena observed in the 'errors'. It is possible that by adding certain predictor variables to the model (part of) the correlation or changing variance over time is 'explained'. Because of this in the literature 'correlated observations' is sometimes followed by 'given the predictor variables in the statistical model'.

4.8 The modelling of time

In the foregoing sections, for both GEE and random coefficient analysis, time was modelled as a continuous variable. A major disadvantage of this

Table 4.4. Example dataset with time as a continuous variable and as a categorical variable with dummy coding

ID	Time (continuous)	Time (categorical)				
		Dummy1	Dummy2	Dummy3	Dummy4	Dummy5
1	1	0	0	0	0	0
1	2	1	0	0	0	0
1	3	0	1	0	0	0
1	4	0	0	1	0	0
1	5	0	0	0	1	0
1	6	0	0	0	0	1
2	1	0	0	0	0	0
2	2	1	0	0	0	0
2	3	0	1	0	0	0
2	4	0	0	1	0	0
2	5	0	0	0	1	0
2	6	0	0	0	0	1
:						

approach is that the development over time of outcome variable Y is modelled as a linear function. This is certainly not always true. It has already been mentioned that one of the possible ways to handle this is to model the development over time as a quadratic, or cubic function, etc. With all this modelling, however, there is still some underlying assumption of the shape of the development over time for outcome variable Y. A very elegant solution is to model time as a categorical variable instead of a continuous one. With time as a categorical variable, the 'real' development over time is modelled, without assuming a certain shape of that relationship. Table 4.4 illustrates part of the example dataset with time as a categorical variable.

It should be taken into account that with time as a categorical variable in a situation with six repeated measurements, five regression parameters must be estimated. In the same situation, with time as a continuous variable and assuming a linear relationship, only one regression coefficient must be estimated. So, modelling time as a categorical variable is only interesting when the number of repeated measurements is low (compared to the number of subjects).

Another limitation of the use of time as a categorical variable is the fact that this is only possible when the time intervals between the repeated

Table 4.5. Example of a dataset with four repeated measurements ($N = 3$) with time as a continuous variable with equal measurement points and time as the actual date of measurement

ID	Time (continuous)	Date (in days)
1	1	0
1	2	20
1	3	45
1	4	100
2	1	0
2	2	30
2	3	40
2	4	80
3	1	0
3	2	25
3	3	50
3	4	70

measurements are the same for each subject. It is obvious that with unequal time intervals between subjects, the dummy coding goes wrong.

In the examples presented in this chapter, each subject was assumed to be measured at the same time-points. Time was simply coded as [1, 2, 3, 4, 5, 6]. However, with both GEE analysis and random coefficient analysis it is possible to model the actual time of each measurement. For instance, the number of days or weeks after a certain baseline measurement can be used as a time indicator (Table 4.5). This is far more realistic, because subjects are almost never measured at exactly the same time. For each subject this indicates that a different time sequence of the measurements is modelled, which directly implies that time cannot be modelled as a categorical variable.

Sections 4.5.4.4 and 4.6.3.2 discussed the results of a longitudinal analysis of the relationships between an outcome variable Y and several predictor variables with unequally spaced time intervals. The results tended to be quite different from the situation in which equally spaced time intervals were considered. These differences were found between two datasets that only differed in the coding of the time variable. It should be noted that if time is used as a categorical variable, this difference does not occur. This is due to the fact that in the dummy coding the real time intervals are no longer included.

Output 4.14. Results of two GEE analyses: one GEE analysis with time as a continuous variable (A), and one GEE analysis with time as a categorical variable (B)

```
(A) Linear Generalized Estimating Equations
Response: YCONT    Corr: Exchangeable
Column   Name           Coeff   StErr   p-value
-----------------------------------------------
     0   Constant       4.058   0.056         0
     2   TIME           0.126   0.011         0
-----------------------------------------------
n:147  s:0.784  #iter:10
Estimate of common correlation 0.595


(B) Linear Generalized Estimating Equations
Response: YCONT    Corr: Exchangeable
Column   Name           Coeff   StErr   p-value
-----------------------------------------------
     0   Constant       4.435   0.055     0.000
     8   TIME1         -0.112   0.038     0.004
     9   TIME2         -0.169   0.044     0.000
    10   TIME3         -0.261   0.046     0.000
    11   TIME4          0.241   0.052     0.000
    12   TIME5          0.691   0.063     0.000
-----------------------------------------------
n:147  s:0.749  #iter:10
Estimate of common correlation 0.674
```

When one is only interested in the relationship with time, this is no problem; the only thing one should worry about then is a correct interpretation of the different dummy variables. However, when one is interested in the relationship with other variables than time, this can lead to major problems in the interpretation of the regression coefficients.

Another problem with the use of dummy variables for the coding of time arises when there are missing observations. In such situations, it is possible that the dummy variable coding does not have the same meaning as it should have for a complete dataset.

4.8.1 Example

Output 4.14 shows the results of a GEE analysis in which the outcome variable Y is related to time as a continuous outcome variable, assuming a linear

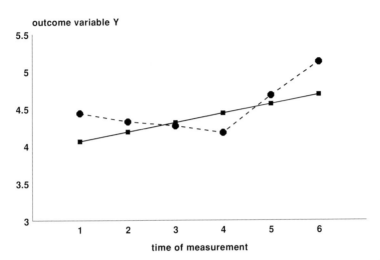

Figure 4.13. The modelled development of outcome variable *Y* over time, estimated with two different GEE analyses (■ —— time continuous, • – – – time categorical).

relationship with time. In the same output, the results of a GEE analysis are shown in which the outcome variable *Y* is related to time as a categorical variable, coded as dummy variables in such a way as has been presented in Table 4.4.

From the first part of the output (4.14(A)) it can be seen that the regression coefficient of time is 0.126, which indicates that there is an increase over time in outcome variable *Y*, and that for an increase in each time unit (i.e. a year) the outcome variable *Y* increases with 0.126 units. The second part of the output (4.14(B)) shows quite a different picture. The regression coefficients of the five dummy variables (there were six measurements in the example dataset, so there are five dummy variables) can be interpreted as follows: compared to the first measurement (which is the reference 'category'), there is a decrease in outcome variable *Y* at the second measurement ($\beta = -0.112$). At the third measurement the decrease continues ($\beta = -0.169$), and at the fourth measurement the lowest point is reached. At the fifth and the sixth measurements the value of outcome variable *Y* is higher than the baseline value, indicating a steep increase during the last two measurements. Figure 4.13 illustrates the results of both models.

It is quite clear that the modelling of time as a categorical variable is much closer to the 'real' observed development over time for outcome variable *Y*.

Output 4.15. Results of two GEE analyses to determine the longitudinal relationship between outcome variable Y and four predictor variables: one with time as a continuous variable (A) and one with time as a categorical variable (B)

```
(A) Linear Generalized Estimating Equations
Response: YCONT    Corr: Exchangeable
Column  Name        Coeff   StErr    p-value
--------------------------------------------
    0   Constant    3.617   0.680    0.000
    2   TIME        0.108   0.014    0.000
    4   X1         -0.024   0.274    0.931
    5   X2          0.111   0.023    0.000
    6   X3         -0.111   0.061    0.069
    7   X4          0.101   0.131    0.440
--------------------------------------------
n:147  s:0.747  #iter:12
Estimate of common correlation 0.562
```

```
(B) Linear Generalized Estimating Equations
Response: YCONT    Corr: Exchangeable
Column  Name        Coeff   StErr    p-value
--------------------------------------------
    0   Constant    3.988   0.688    0.000
    4   X1         -0.029   0.276    0.918
    5   X2          0.103   0.019    0.000
    6   X3         -0.084   0.054    0.117
    7   X4          0.111   0.130    0.393
    8   TIME1      -0.118   0.038    0.002
    9   TIME2      -0.190   0.045    0.000
   10   TIME3      -0.299   0.047    0.000
   11   TIME4       0.154   0.059    0.009
   12   TIME5       0.620   0.070    0.000
--------------------------------------------
n:147  s:0.711  #iter:12
Estimate of common correlation 0.646
```

The following step is to investigate the consequences of the different ways of modelling time for the magnitude of the regression coefficients reflecting the longitudinal relationship with other variables. Therefore both time indicators were used in the analysis of the longitudinal relationship between the outcome variable Y and the four predictor variables X_1 to X_4. Output 4.15 shows the results of these two GEE analyses. From Output 4.15 it can be seen that there are some differences between the two analyses, but that these differences are only marginal.

To summarize, when one is interested in the development over time of a particular outcome variable, when the number of repeated measurements is not very large, when the repeated measurements are equally spaced between subjects, and when there are no missing observations, it is highly recommended that time should be modelled as a categorical variable. In all other situations, it is more appropriate to model time as a continuous variable.

Other possibilities for modelling longitudinal data

5.1 Introduction

In Chapter 4, GEE analysis and random coefficient analysis were introduced as two (sophisticated) methods that can be used to analyse the longitudinal relationship between an outcome variable Y and several predictor variables. In this chapter, the models described in Chapter 4 (which are known as standard or marginal models) are slightly altered in order to answer specific research questions.

5.2 Alternative models

5.2.1 Time-lag model

It is assumed that the greatest advantage of a longitudinal study design in epidemiological research is that causal relationships can be detected. However, in fact this is only partly true for experimental designs (see Chapter 9). In observational longitudinal studies in general, no answer can be given to the question of whether a certain relationship is causal or not. With the standard or marginal models already described in Chapter 4, it is only possible to detect associations between an outcome variable Y and one (or more) predictor variable(s) X. When there is some rationale about possible causation in observational longitudinal studies, these associations are called 'quasi-causal relationships'. In every epidemiological textbook a list of arguments can be found which can give an indication as to whether or not an observed relationship is causal (see Table 1.1). One of these concerns the temporal sequence of the relationship. When the predictor variable X precedes the outcome variable Y, the observed relationship may be causal (Figure 5.1).

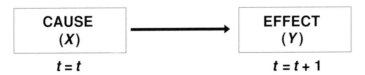

Figure 5.1. Temporal sequence between predictor variable (cause) and outcome variable (effect).

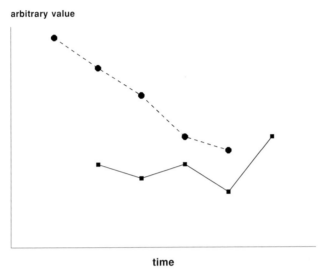

Figure 5.2. Illustration of the time-lag model; predictor variable X is modelled prior to the outcome variable Y (■ —— outcome variable, • - - - predictor variable).

With a small change in the standard models described in Chapter 4, this time sequence between predictor variables X and outcome variable Y can be modelled. In this so-called time-lag model the predictor variables X are modelled prior in time to the outcome variable Y (Figure 5.2). The corresponding equation is:

$$Y_{it} = \beta_0 + \sum_{j=1}^{J} \beta_{1j} X_{ijt-1} + \cdots \tag{5.1}$$

where Y_{it} are observations for subject i at time t, β_0 is the intercept, X_{ijt-1} is the independent variable j for subject i at time $t-1$, β_{1j} is the regression coefficient for independent variable j, and J is the number of independent variables.

In a time-lag model the predictor variables X at time-point $t - 1$ are related to the outcome variable Y at time-point t. The remaining part of the model is equivalent to the standard model described in Chapter 4 (see Equation (4.3)).

Both the time-lag model and the standard model pool together longitudinal and cross-sectional relationships into one regression coefficient. This is sometimes hard to understand, but it indicates that both the relationships between absolute values at each time-point ('between-subjects' relationships) and the relationships between changes between subsequent time-points ('within-subject' relationships) are used to estimate the overall regression coefficients (see Section 4.5.3). The only difference between the time-lag model and the standard model is that the time-lag model takes into account the temporal sequence of a possible cause and effect. The question then arises: should a time-lag model be used in every situation in which a causal relationship is suspected? The answer is no! In fact, a time-lag model can only be useful when the time periods between subsequent measurements are short. When the time periods are long, the biological plausibility of a time lag between predictor variable X and outcome variable Y is not very clear. Furthermore, sometimes a time lag is already taken into account in the way a certain predictor variable is measured. For instance, when a lifestyle parameter such as dietary intake or physical inactivity is used as predictor variable in relation to some sort of disease outcome, both lifestyle parameters are often measured by some method of retrospective recall (e.g. measurement of the average amount of dietary intake of a certain nutrient over the previous three months). In other words, when a time lag is included in the method of measuring the predictor variable X, a statistical time-lag model is not very appropriate. In general, the usefulness of a time-lag model depends on the biological plausibility of a time lag in the relationship analysed.

It is also possible that the results of a time-lag model are a reflection of the results that would have been found in a standard model. This occurs when the relative stability (see Chapter 11) of both the outcome variable and the predictor variable of interest is rather high. In fact, the standard/marginal relationships carry over to the time-lag relationship through the relative stability of the variables involved in the relationship investigated. Figure 5.3 illustrates this phenomenon.

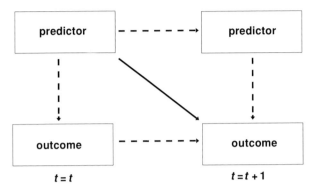

Figure 5.3. A time-lag relationship can be a reflection of the standard relationship when the relative stability of both the outcome variable and the predictor variable is high.

5.2.2 Modelling of changes

As mentioned before, both the standard model and the time-lag model pool together 'between-subjects' and 'within-subject' relationships. Although this is an important strength of the analysis, it also limits the interpretation of the results in such a way that no separation can be made between the two aspects of longitudinal relationships. This can be a problem especially when the variation in absolute values between subjects exceeds the changes over time within subjects. In this particular situation, in the pooled analysis the longitudinal within-subject relationships will be more or less overruled by the cross-sectional between-subjects relationships (see Figure 5.4). This problem arises in particular when the time periods between subsequent measurements are relatively short, or when there is a strong (mostly non-observable) influence from the background variables (see Section 5.4).

Because of this limitation of both the standard model and the time-lag model, a model can be used in which the cross-sectional part is more or less 'removed' from the analysis. One possibility is not to model absolute values at each time-point, but to model changes between two consecutive measurements of both the outcome variable Y and the predictor variables X (Figure 5.5). The corresponding equation is:

$$(Y_{it} - Y_{it-1}) = \beta_0 + \sum_{j=1}^{J} \beta_{1j}(X_{ijt} - X_{ijt-1}) + \cdots \tag{5.2}$$

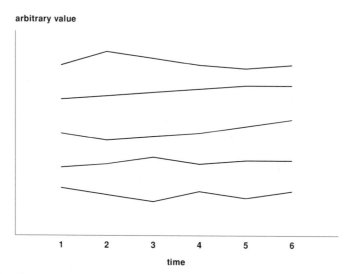

arbitrary value

Figure 5.4. Illustration of a longitudinal study in which the changes over time within one subject are less than the differences between subjects; the cross-sectional relationships will 'overrule' the longitudinal relationships.

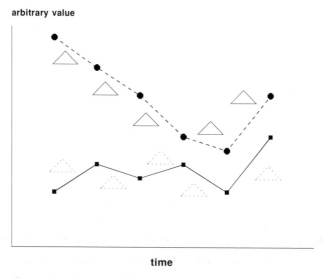

arbitrary value

Figure 5.5. Illustration of the modelling of changes; changes in predictor variable X are related to changes in the outcome variable Y (■ —— outcome variable, • - - - predictor variable).

where Y_{it} are observations for subject i at time t, Y_{it-1} is the observation for subject i at time $t - 1$, β_0 is the intercept, X_{ijt} is the independent variable j for subject i at time t, X_{ijt-1} is the independent variable j for subject i at time $t - 1$, β_{1j} is the regression coefficient for independent variable j, and J is the number of independent variables.

The remaining part of the model can be the same as in the standard model, but the changes for the time-dependent covariates can also be modelled. The modelling of changes looks quite simple, but it can be very complicated, owing to the difficulty of defining changes between subsequent measurements (see Chapter 8).

5.2.3 Autoregressive model

Another way in which to 'remove' the cross-sectional part of the relationships is to use an autoregressive model. Autoregressive models are also known as Markov models, conditional models or transition models, and an extensive amount of literature has been devoted to these types of models (Rosner et al., 1985; Rosner and Munoz, 1988; Zeger and Qaqish, 1988; Stanek et al., 1989; Lindsey, 1993). The corresponding equation is:

$$Y_{it} = \beta_0 + \sum_{j=1}^{J} \beta_{1j} X_{ijt-1} + \beta_2 Y_{it-1} + \cdots \tag{5.3}$$

where Y_{it} are observations for subject i at time t, β_0 is the intercept, X_{ijt-1} is the independent variable j for subject i at time $t - 1$, β_{1j} is the regression coefficient for independent variable j, J is the number of independent variables, Y_{it-1} is the observation for subject i at time $t - 1$, and β_2 is the autoregression coefficient.

In an autoregressive model the value of the outcome variable Y at time-point t is related not only to the value of the predictor variable X at time-point $t - 1$, but also to the value of the outcome variable Y at $t - 1$. The remaining part of the model is usually the same as in the standard model. The model shown in Equation (5.3) is called a 'first-order' autoregressive model, because the outcome variable Y at time-point t is only related to the value of the outcome variable Y at $t - 1$. In a 'second-order' or 'third-order' autoregressive model, the outcome variable Y at time-point t is also related to the value of the standard model:

$$
\begin{bmatrix} Y_1 \\ Y_2 \\ Y_3 \\ Y_4 \\ Y_5 \\ Y_6 \end{bmatrix} = \beta_0 + \beta_1 \begin{bmatrix} X_1 \\ X_2 \\ X_3 \\ X_4 \\ X_5 \\ X_6 \end{bmatrix} + \ldots
$$

time-lag model:

$$
\begin{bmatrix} Y_2 \\ Y_3 \\ Y_4 \\ Y_5 \\ Y_6 \end{bmatrix} = \beta_0 + \beta_1 \begin{bmatrix} X_1 \\ X_2 \\ X_3 \\ X_4 \\ X_5 \end{bmatrix} + \ldots
$$

modelling of changes:

$$
\begin{bmatrix} Y_2 - Y_1 \\ Y_3 - Y_2 \\ Y_4 - Y_3 \\ Y_5 - Y_4 \\ Y_6 - Y_5 \end{bmatrix} = \beta_0 + \beta_1 \begin{bmatrix} X_2 - X_1 \\ X_3 - X_2 \\ X_4 - X_3 \\ X_5 - X_4 \\ X_6 - X_5 \end{bmatrix} + \ldots
$$

autoregressive model:

$$
\begin{bmatrix} Y_2 \\ Y_3 \\ Y_4 \\ Y_5 \\ Y_6 \end{bmatrix} = \beta_0 + \beta_1 \begin{bmatrix} X_1 \\ X_2 \\ X_3 \\ X_4 \\ X_5 \end{bmatrix} + \beta_2 \begin{bmatrix} Y_1 \\ Y_2 \\ Y_3 \\ Y_4 \\ Y_5 \end{bmatrix} + \ldots
$$

Figure 5.6. Overview of different models used to analyse the longitudinal relationship between an outcome variable *Y* and a predictor variable *X*.

outcome variable Y at $t - 2$ or $t - 3$. The idea underlying the autoregressive model is that the value of an outcome variable at each time-point is primarily influenced by the value of this variable one measurement earlier. To estimate the 'real' influence of the predictor variables on the outcome variable, the model should therefore correct for the value of the outcome variable at time-point $t - 1$.

5.2.4 Overview

Figure 5.6 gives an overview of the way in which the regression coefficients of interest relate the development of a particular predictor variable X to the development of an outcome variable Y in the different (alternative) models used to analyse longitudinal data. It should be noted that, like the standard model, all alternative models can also be modelled with random coefficients.

5.2.5 Example
5.2.5.1 Introduction

In the following example the results of the three mentioned alternative models will be compared to the standard model (described in Chapter 4). For all three models both GEE analysis and random coefficient analysis will be used to estimate the regression coefficients. When GEE is used a correction is made for the within-subjects correlations by assuming a certain 'working correlation structure'. It was argued that the choice of a particular structure can be based on the observed within-subject correlations of the outcome variable Y. When the longitudinal analysis is limited to the 'within-subject' relationships (i.e. modelling of changes and the autoregressive model), the correction for the within-subject correlations is somewhat different than for the standard model. When changes are modelled, the within-subject correlations between the changes are in general much lower than the within-subject correlations of the 'absolute' values. The same is true for the autoregressive model. The latter is perhaps a bit difficult to understand, but it has to do with the fact that in GEE analysis a correction is made for the 'correlated errors', rather than for the correlated 'observations'. Although this is basically the same, in an autoregressive model part of the correlations in the observations is 'explained' by the addition of the outcome variable Y at $t - 1$ to the model. In an autoregressive model, the within-subject correlations of the 'errors' are therefore different from the within-subject correlations of the 'observations'. In fact, in both the modelling of changes and the autoregressive model, correction for the within-subject correlations is part of the model. In those situations, an independent correlation structure will (often) be the most appropriate choice.

In the modelling of changes yet another problem arises, because changes between subsequent measurements can be defined in many different ways (see Chapter 8). In the following examples the changes are defined as the absolute change between subsequent measurements.

5.2.5.2 *Data structure for alternative models*

There is no statistical software available which is capable of performing one of the alternative models automatically. For the alternative modelling of longitudinal data, the dataset has to be reconstructed so that the standard software can be used for either GEE analysis or random coefficient analysis. The way in which the data should be reconstructed is illustrated in Figure 5.7.

5.2.5.3 *GEE analysis*

The output of the GEE analysis, used to answer the question of whether there is a longitudinal relationship between outcome variable Y and the predictor

standard model

ID	Y	X_1	time
1	3.5	1.53	1
1	3.7	1.43	2
1	3.9	2.01	3
1	3.0	2.22	4
1	3.2	2.12	5
1	3.2	1.95	6
2	4.1	2.00	1
2	4.1	2.30	2
⋮			
N	5.0	1.78	5
N	4.7	1.99	6

time-lag model

ID	Y	X_1	time
1	3.7	1.53	2
1	3.9	1.43	3
1	3.0	2.01	4
1	3.2	2.22	5
1	3.2	2.12	6
2	4.2	2.00	2
⋮			
N	4.7	1.78	6

modelling of changes

ID	$Y_t - Y_{t-1}$	$X_t - X_{t-1}$	time
1	−0.2	0.10	1
1	−0.2	−0.58	2
1	0.9	−0.20	3
1	−0.2	0.10	4
1	0.0	0.17	5
2	−0.1	−0.30	1
⋮			
N	0.3	−0.21	5

autoregressive model

ID	Y	Y_{t-1}	X_1	time
1	3.7	3.5	1.43	2
1	3.9	3.7	2.01	3
1	3.0	3.9	2.22	4
1	3.2	3.0	2.12	5
1	3.2	3.2	1.95	6
2	4.2	4.1	2.30	2
⋮				
N	4.7	5.0	1.99	6

Figure 5.7. Data structures for various models used to analyse longitudinal relationships.

variables X_1 to X_4 and time, based on alternative longitudinal models is shown in Output 5.1 (time-lag model), Output 5.2 (modelling of changes) and Output 5.3 (autoregressive model).

In addition to the changes in outcome variable Y, in the modelling of changes, the changes in the predictor variable X_2 are added to the model. For all other predictor variables the absolute values, either at baseline (for the time-independent predictor variables X_1 and X_4) or at the start of the time period over which the changes are calculated (for the time-dependent predictor variable X_3), are added to the model. Furthermore, from Output 5.2 it can be seen that an independent correlation structure has been chosen as 'working correlation structure'. Therefore, the last line of the output, which provides the estimation of the common correlation, is lacking.

Output 5.1. Results of a GEE analysis with
a time-lag model

```
Linear Generalized Estimating Equations
Response: YCONT    Corr: Exchangeable
Column  Name       Coeff  StErr  p-value
----------------------------------------
     0  Constant   2.883  0.719  0.000
     2  TIME       0.156  0.017  0.000
     4  X1         0.123  0.287  0.668
     5  X2         0.151  0.031  0.000
     6  X3         0.097  0.070  0.164
     7  X4         0.128  0.130  0.323
----------------------------------------
n:147   s:0.733   #iter:12
Estimate of common correlation 0.577
```

Output 5.2. Results of a GEE analysis with
modelling of changes

```
Linear Generalized Estimating Equations
Response: DELY     Corr: Independence
Column  Name       Coeff   StErr  p-value
----------------------------------------
     0  Constant  -0.615   0.182  0.001
     2  TIME       0.161   0.013  0.000
     4  X1         0.059   0.076  0.431
     5  DELX2      0.084   0.025  0.001
     6  X3         0.118   0.056  0.036
     7  X4         0.077   0.031  0.015
----------------------------------------
n:147   s:0.529   #iter:12
```

As for the modelling of changes, an independent correlation structure is also chosen for the autoregressive model (Output 5.3). Moreover, in the output a new predictor variable is present (YCONTPRE). This predictor variable is the value of outcome variable Y measured one time-point earlier (see explanation of the autoregressive model in Section 5.2.3). From the output it can be seen that the value of Y at $t - 1$ is highly positively related

Output 5.3. Results of a GEE analysis with an autoregressive model

```
Linear Generalized Estimating Equations
Response: YCONT    Corr: Independence
Column  Name       Coeff   StErr   p-value
-------------------------------------------
     0  Constant  -0.125   0.251     0.619
     2  TIME       0.154   0.013     0.000
     4  X1         0.139   0.096     0.149
     5  X2         0.091   0.014     0.000
     6  X3         0.012   0.048     0.802
     7  X4         0.027   0.043     0.531
     8  YCONTPRE   0.767   0.025     0.000
-------------------------------------------
   n:147   s:0.506   #iter:12
```

Table 5.1. Regression coefficients and standard errors regarding the longitudinal relationship (estimated by GEE analysis) between outcome variable Y and several predictor variables (X_1 to X_4 and time); the standard or marginal model compared to alternative models

	Standard model	Time-lag model	Modelling of changes	Autoregressive model
X_1	−0.02 (0.27)	0.12 (0.29)	0.06 (0.07)	0.14 (0.10)
X_2	0.11 (0.02)	0.15 (0.03)	0.08 (0.03)	0.09 (0.01)
X_3	−0.11 (0.06)	0.10 (0.07)	0.12 (0.06)	0.01 (0.05)
X_4	0.01 (0.13)	0.13 (0.13)	0.08 (0.03)	0.03 (0.04)
Time	0.11 (0.01)	0.16 (0.02)	0.16 (0.01)	0.15 (0.01)

to the development of outcome variable Y, which is of course not really surprising. The regression coefficient of the predictor variable YCONTPRE is also known as the autoregression coefficient. In Table 5.1 the results of the different GEE analyses are summarized.

5.2.5.4 Random coefficient analysis

The output of a random coefficient analysis to answer the question of whether there is a longitudinal relationship between outcome variable Y and the predictor variables X_1 to X_4 and time, based on alternative longitudinal models, is shown in Output 5.4 (time-lag model), Output 5.5 (modelling of changes) and Output 5.6 (autoregressive model). The predictor variables in the random coefficient analysis were modelled in the same way as has been described for the corresponding GEE analysis.

Output 5.4. Results of a random coefficient analysis with a time-lag model

```
log likelihood = -640.37118
-------------------------------------------------------------------------------
ycont        Coeff    Std. Err.       z     P > |z|    [95% Conf.   Interval]
-------------------------------------------------------------------------------
time     0.1582593    0.01579    10.023    0.000     0.1273114    0.1892072
  x1     0.100344     0.2783983    0.360    0.719    -0.4453067    0.6459947
  x2     0.1406945    0.0248505    5.662    0.000     0.0919884    0.1894006
  x3     0.0958463    0.0662912    1.446    0.148    -0.034082     0.2257746
  x4     0.1318902    0.1204924    1.095    0.274    -0.1042707    0.368051
_cons    2.948436     0.677334     4.353    0.000     1.620886     4.275986
-------------------------------------------------------------------------------

Variance at level 1
-------------------------------------------------------------------------------
0.20557651  (0.01383197)

Variances and covariances of random effects
-------------------------------------------------------------------------------
***level 2 (id)
  var(1):   0.29172121  (0.08177964)
cov(1,2):  -0.01191011  (0.01513772)  cor(1,2):  -0.25634858
  var(2):   0.00739949  (0.00364189)
```

From the output of both the modelling of changes and the autoregressive model, it can be seen that both the variance of the random intercept and the variance of the random slope are close to zero, although for the modelling of changes this is far more pronounced than for the autoregressive model. So, assuming a random intercept and a random slope in the longitudinal random coefficient model is not really necessary. In fact, this finding is comparable to the fact that in the GEE analysis for these two alternative models an independent correlation structure is considered to be the most appropriate choice for a 'working correlation structure'. In Table 5.2 the results of the different random coefficient analyses are summarized.

Output 5.5. Results of a random coefficient analysis with modelling of changes

```
log likelihood = -571.64658
---------------------------------------------------------------------------
  dely       Coeff   Std. Err.        z     P > |z|   [95% Conf.    Interval]
---------------------------------------------------------------------------
  time    0.1613603   0.0143233   11.266    0.000     0.1332871    0.1894334
    x1    0.0594099   0.109767     0.541    0.588    -0.1557295    0.2745492
 delx2    0.0842789   0.020463     4.119    0.000     0.0441722    0.1243857
    x3    0.1178238   0.0569115    2.070    0.038     0.0062793    0.2293684
    x4    0.0769342   0.0474924    1.620    0.105    -0.0161492    0.1700175
 _cons   -0.6151973   0.2684902   -2.291    0.022    -1.141428    -0.0889663
---------------------------------------------------------------------------

Variance at level 1
---------------------------------------------------------------------------
0.27737764 (0.01446915)

Variances and covariances of random effects
---------------------------------------------------------------------------
***level 2 (id)

  var(1):   7.729 × 10⁻¹⁰  (0.00002627)
cov(1,2):  -3.125 × 10⁻¹⁰  (0.0000106)    cor(1,2): -1
  var(2):   1.263 × 10⁻¹⁰  (4.280 × 10⁻⁶)
```

5.3 Comments

Although the magnitude of the regression coefficients for the different models cannot be interpreted in the same way, a comparison between the regression coefficients and standard errors shows directly that the results are quite different. Using an alternative model can lead to different conclusions than when using the standard model. On the one hand this is strange, because all analyses attempt to answer the question of whether there is a relationship between outcome variable Y and the four predictor variables and time. On the other hand, however, with the four models, different parts of the longitudinal relationships are analysed, and the results of the models should be interpreted in different ways. To obtain the most general answer to the question of whether there is a longitudinal relationship between the outcome variable Y and the four predictor variables and time, the results of several models should be combined (Twisk, 1997). In practice, however, this almost never happens: a priori the most appropriate model is chosen (usually the 'standard' model), and only those results are reported.

Output 5.6. Results of a random coefficient analysis with an autoregressive model

```
log likelihood = -538.88027
-----------------------------------------------------------------------------
    ycont     Coeff   Std. Err.       z    P > |z|   [95% Conf.   Interval]
-----------------------------------------------------------------------------
     time   0.1544628  0.0141067   10.950   0.000    0.1268142   0.1821114
       x1   0.1319348  0.1086507    1.214   0.225   -0.0810165   0.3448862
       x2   0.090171   0.0148155    6.086   0.000    0.0611331   0.1192089
       x3   0.0077988  0.0486855    0.160   0.873   -0.0876232   0.1032207
       x4   0.0317883  0.0491346    0.647   0.518   -1.0645138   0.1280903
  ycontpre  0.760324   0.0291116   26.118   0.000    0.7032664   0.8173816
    _cons  -0.0883166  0.2944095   -0.300   0.764   -0.6653485   0.4887154
-----------------------------------------------------------------------------
Variance at level 1
-----------------------------------------------------------------------------
0.2483483 (0.01470989)

Variances and covariances of random effects
-----------------------------------------------------------------------------
***level 2 (id)
  var(1):   0.0134973   (0.02323551)
cov(1,2):  -0.00475411  (0.00739352)   cor(1,2): -1
  var(2):   0.00167453  (0.00239752)
```

Table 5.2. Regression coefficients and standard errors regarding the longitudinal relationship (estimated by random coefficient analysis) between outcome variable Y and several predictor variables (X_1 to X_4 and time); the standard or marginal model compared to alternative models

	Standard model	Time-lag model	Modelling of changes	Autoregressive model
X_1	−0.01 (0.27)	0.10 (0.28)	0.06 (0.11)	0.13 (0.11)
X_2	0.11 (0.02)	0.14 (0.02)	0.08 (0.02)	0.09 (0.01)
X_3	−0.12 (0.06)	0.10 (0.07)	0.11 (0.06)	0.01 (0.05)
X_4	0.04 (0.12)	0.13 (0.12)	0.08 (0.05)	0.03 (0.05)
Time	0.11 (0.01)	0.16 (0.02)	0.16 (0.01)	0.15 (0.01)

In Chapter 4 it has already been mentioned that GEE analyses do not give reliable information about the 'fit' of the statistical model, whereas with random coefficient analysis, likelihood values can be obtained. However, when deciding which model should be used to obtain the best answer to a particular research question, comparing the 'fit' of the models will not provide much interesting information. First of all, only the time-lag model and the autoregressive model can be directly compared to each other, because the autoregressive model can be seen as an extension of the time-lag model. The modelling of changes is totally different, while in the standard model more observations are used than in the alternative models. The problem is that the number of observations highly influences the likelihood of each specific statistical model. Looking at the fit of the models, it is obvious for instance that the autoregressive model provides a much better fit than the time-lag model. This is due to the fact that a high percentage of variance of the outcome variable Y at time-point t is explained by the value of the outcome variable Y at $t - 1$. This can be seen from the values of the scale parameter (s) presented in the GEE output and the log likelihood presented in the output of the random coefficient analysis. Both values are much lower in the autoregressive model than in the time-lag model. This does not mean that the autoregressive model should be used to obtain the best answer to the question of whether there is a longitudinal relationship between outcome variable Y and one (or more) predictor variable(s) X. In general, it should be realized that it is better to base the choice of a specific longitudinal model on logical considerations instead of statistical ones. If, for instance, it is expected that a predictor variable measured at time-point t will influence the outcome variable at time-point $t + 1$, then a time-lag model is suitable. If, however, it is expected that the predictor and outcome variables are more directly related, a time-lag model is not suitable, and so forth.

As with the standard model discussed in Chapter 4, in order to simplify the discussion the models presented in Chapter 5 were all simple linear models: no squared terms, no complicated relationships with time, no difficult interactions, etc. Furthermore, in the explanation of the various alternative models it was mentioned that the remaining parts of the models were the same as the standard model. This is not necessarily true. It is also possible to combine different models with each other. For instance, in the autoregressive model (Equation (5.3)) the outcome variable at time-point t (Y_{it}) was related to the predictor variable at time-point $t - 1$ (X_{it-1}), corrected for the value of the outcome variable at $t - 1$ (Y_{it-1}). It is, however, possible to remove the time lag from this model, by using the value of the predictor variable at t, instead of its value at time-point $t - 1$. It must be stressed, however, that the choice of possible combinations of different models must also be based on logical considerations and on the research questions to be answered.

It has already been mentioned that with the modelling of changes and with the autoregressive model the between-subject part of the analysis is more or less removed from the analysis. With both models only the longitudinal relationships are analysed. It is therefore surprising that the results of the longitudinal analyses with the modelling of changes and the autoregressive model are quite different (see Tables 5.1 and 5.2). One reason for the difference in results is that both alternative models use a different model of change. This can be explained by assuming a longitudinal study with just two measurements. In the autoregressive model, $Y_2 = \beta_0 + \beta_1 Y_1$, while in the modelling of changes, $Y_2 - Y_1 = \beta_0$ (where β_0 is the absolute change between subsequent measurements), which is equal to $Y_2 = \beta_0 + Y_1$. The difference between the two equations is the coefficient β_1. In the modelling of changes the 'change' is a fixed parameter, while in the autoregressive model the 'change' is a function of the value of Y_1 (for a detailed explanation of this phenomenon, see Chapter 8). Another reason for the differences in results between the modelling of changes and the autoregressive model is the different modelling of the predictor variables. It has already been mentioned that for the modelling of changes the changes in the predictor variables were also modelled. In the autoregressive model, however, the predictor variables measured at $t - 1$ were used. It is obvious that different modelling of the predictor variables can lead to different results. To illustrate this, Output 5.7 shows the results of an autoregressive model, in which the predictor variables are modelled in the same way as has been described for the modelling of changes.

From Output 5.7 it can be seen that (as expected) the results of an autoregressive model with the predictor variables modelled as changes are closer to the results of the modelling of changes than when the predictor variables were modelled at $t - 1$. The most important message which emerges is that the modelling of the predictor variables can highly influence the results of the longitudinal analyses performed with alternative models. In other words, one should be very careful in the interpretation of the regression coefficients derived from such models.

Output 5.7. Results of a GEE analysis with an autoregressive model, in which the predictor variables are modelled in the same way as in the modelling of changes

```
Linear Generalized Estimating Equations
Response: YCONT          Corr: Independence
Column    Name           Coeff    StErr    p-value
-------------------------------------------------
    0     Constant        0.262    0.258    0.310
    2     TIME            0.174    0.013    0.000
    4     X1             -0.005    0.101    0.964
    5     DELX2           0.063    0.024    0.010
    6     X3              0.028    0.048    0.565
    7     X4              0.115    0.042    0.006
    8     YCONTPRE        0.810    0.022    0.000
-------------------------------------------------
n:147  s:0.516  #iter:11
```

Table 5.3. Standardized regression coefficients and 95% confidence intervals (calculated with GEE analysis) regarding the longitudinal relationship between lung function parameters (forced vital capacity (FVC) and the forced expiratory volume in one second (FEV1)) and smoking behaviour; a comparison between the standard model and the modelling of changes

	FVC	FEV1
Standard model	−0.03 (−0.11 to 0.06)	−0.01 (−0.09 to 0.06)
Modelling of changes	−0.13 (−0.22 to −0.04)**	−0.14 (−0.25 to −0.04)**

** $p < 0.01$.

5.4 Another example

One of the most striking examples to illustrate the necessity of using information from different models has been given in a study also based on data from the Amsterdam Growth and Health Longitudinal Study (Twisk et al., 1998a). The purpose of that study was to investigate the relationship between smoking behaviour and the development of two lung function parameters: forced vital capacity (FVC) and forced expiratory volume in one second (FEV1). Although the results of the standard model did not show any relationship between smoking behaviour and the development of lung function parameters, the modelling of changes revealed a strong negative relationship between smoking behaviour and the development of both lung function parameters (see Table 5.3). So, although the absolute values of the lung function parameters were not influenced by smoking behaviour, the changes in lung function parameters over time were highly influenced by smoking behaviour. This study is a nice example of the situation illustrated earlier in Figure 5.4.

Dichotomous outcome variables

6.1 Simple methods

6.1.1 Two measurements

When a dichotomous outcome variable is measured twice over time in the same subjects, a 2×2 table can be constructed as shown below (where n stands for the number of subjects and p stands for a proportion of the total number of subjects N).

		t_2		
		1	2	Total
t_1	1	$n_{11}(p_{11})$	$n_{12}(p_{12})$	$n_{1(t1)}(p_{1(t1)})$
	2	$n_{21}(p_{21})$	$n_{22}(p_{22})$	$n_{2(t1)}(p_{2(t1)})$
	Total	$n_{1(t2)}(p_{1(t2)})$	$n_{2(t2)}(p_{2(t2)})$	$N(1)$

The simplest way to estimate the development over time is to compare the proportion of subjects in group 1 at $t_1(p_{1(t1)})$ with the proportion of subjects in group 1 at $t_2(p_{1(t2)})$. The difference in proportions is calculated as $(p_{1(t2)} - p_{1(t1)})$, and Equation (6.1) shows how to calculate the corresponding standard error:

$$SE(p_{1(t2)} - p_{1(t1)}) = \frac{\sqrt{n_{1(t2)} + n_{1(t1)}}}{N} \tag{6.1}$$

where SE is the standard error, $p_{1(t2)}$ is the proportion of subjects in group 1 at $t = 2$, $p_{1(t1)}$ is the proportion of subjects in group 1 at $t = 1$, $n_{1(t2)}$ is the number of subjects in group 1 at $t = 2$, $n_{1(t1)}$ is the number of subjects in group 1 at $t = 1$, and N is the total number of subjects.

The 95% confidence interval for the difference (difference ± 1.96 times the standard error) is used to answer the question of whether there is a significant change over time. The problem with the difference in proportions is that it basically provides an indication of the difference between the changes in opposite directions. If all subjects from group 1 at $t = 1$ move to group 2 at $t = 2$, and all subjects from group 2 at $t = 1$ move to group 1 at $t = 2$, the difference in proportions reveals no changes over time.

A widely used method to determine whether there is a change over time in a dichotomous outcome variable is the McNemar test. This is an alternative χ^2 test, which takes into account the fact that the observed proportions in the 2×2 table are not independent. The McNemar test is, in principle, based on the difference between n_{12} and n_{21}, and the test statistic follows a χ^2 distribution with one degree of freedom (Equation (6.2)).

$$\chi^2 = \frac{(n_{12} - n_{21} - 1)^2}{n_{12} + n_{21}} \tag{6.2}$$

where n_{12} is the number of subjects in group 1 at $t = 1$ and in group 2 at $t = 2$, and n_{21} is the number of subjects in group 2 at $t = 1$ and in group 1 at $t = 2$.

The McNemar test determines whether the change in one direction is equal to the change in another direction. So the McNemar test has the same disadvantages as have been mentioned above for the difference in proportions. It tests the difference between the changes in opposite directions.

A possible way in which to estimate the **total** change over time is to calculate the proportion of subjects who change from one group to another: i.e. $p_{12} + p_{21}$. This 'proportion of change' can be tested for significance by means of the 95% confidence interval (± 1.96 times the standard error). The standard error of this proportion is calculated as:

$$\text{SE}(p_{\text{change}}) = \sqrt{\frac{p_{\text{change}} - (1 - p_{\text{change}})}{N}} \tag{6.3}$$

where SE is the standard error, p_{change} is the 'proportion of change' equal to $p_{12} + p_{21}$, and N is the total number of subjects.

If one is only interested in the proportion of subjects who change in a certain direction (i.e. only a 'decrease' or 'increase' over time) the same procedure can be followed for separate changes. In this respect, a 'proportion of increase' equal to p_{12} or a 'proportion of decrease' equal to p_{21} can be calculated and a 95% confidence interval can be constructed, based on the standard error calculated with Equation (6.3).

It should be noted that when all individuals belong to the same group at baseline, the estimate of the change in opposite directions is equal to the estimate of the total change over time. In that situation, which often occurs in experimental studies, all methods discussed so far can be used to estimate the change over time in a dichotomous outcome variable.

6.1.2 More than two measurements

When more than two measurements are performed on the same subjects, the multivariate extension of the McNemar test can be used. This multivariate extension is known as Cochran's Q, and it has the same disadvantages as the McNemar test. It is a measure of the difference between changes in opposite directions, while in longitudinal studies one is generally interested in the total change over time. To analyse the total change over time, the 'proportion of change' can be calculated in the same way as in the situation with two measurements. To do this, $(T-1)$ 2×2 tables must first be constructed (for $t=1$ and $t=2$, for $t=2$ and $t=3$, and so on). The next step is to calculate the 'proportion of change' for each 2×2 table. To calculate the total proportion of change, Equation (6.4) can be applied:

$$\bar{p} = \frac{1}{N(T-1)} \sum_{i=1}^{N} c_i \qquad (6.4)$$

where $\bar{p}$ is the total 'proportion of change', N is the number of subjects, T is the number of measurements, and c_i is the the number of changes for individual i over time.

6.1.3 Comparing groups

To compare the development over time between two groups, for a dichotomous outcome variable the 'proportion of change' in the two groups can be compared. This can be done by applying the test for two independent proportions: $(p_{g1} - p_{g2})$. The standard error of this difference (needed to create a 95% confidence interval and for testing whether there is a significant difference between the two groups) is calculated by Equation (6.5):

$$\text{SE}(p_{g1} - p_{g2}) = \sqrt{\left[\frac{p_{g1}(1 - p_{g1})}{N_{g1}}\right] + \left[\frac{p_{g2}(1 - p_{g2})}{N_{g2}}\right]} \tag{6.5}$$

where SE is the standard error, p_{g1} is the 'proportion of change' in group 1, p_{g2} is the 'proportion of change' in group 2, N_{g1} is the number of subjects in group 1, and N_{g2} is the number of subjects in group 2.

Of course, this procedure can also be carried out to determine the 'proportion of change' in a certain direction (i.e. the 'proportion of increase' or the 'proportion of decrease'). It should be realized that the calculation of the 'proportion of change' over a particular time period is primarily useful for the longitudinal analysis of datasets with only two measurements. For more information on the analysis of proportions and differences in proportions, reference is made to the classical work of Fleiss (1981).

6.1.4 Example

6.1.4.1 Introduction

The dataset used to illustrate longitudinal analysis with a dichotomous outcome variable is the same as that used to illustrate longitudinal analysis with continuous outcome variables. The only difference is that the outcome variable Y is dichotomized (Y_{dich}). This is done by means of the 66th percentile. At each of the repeated measurements the upper 33% are coded as '1', and the lower 66% are coded as '0' (see Section 1.4).

6.1.4.2 Development over time

To analyse the development of a dichotomous outcome variable Y_{dich} over time, the situation with two measurements will first be illustrated. From the example dataset the first ($t = 1$) and the last ($t = 6$) measurements will be considered. Let us first investigate the 2×2 table, which is presented in Output 6.1.

Because the dichotomization of outcome variable Y_{dich} was based on a fixed value (the 66th percentile), it is **defined** that there is no difference between the changes over time in opposite directions. The proportion of subjects in group 1 at $t = 1$ (33.3%) is almost equal to the proportion of subjects

Output 6.1. 2 x 2 table indicating the relationship between the outcome variable Y_{dich} at $t = 1$ and $t = 6$

```
YDICHT1 OUTCOME VARIABLE Y AT T1 (2 GROUPS)
by YDICHT6 OUTCOME VARIABLE Y AT T6 (2 GROUPS)

                        YDICHT6
              Count
                                           Row
                        0.00      1.00     Total
YDICHT1
              0.00       80        17        97
                                           66.0
              1.00       18        32        50
                                           34.0
            Column       98        49       147
            Total       66.7      33.3     100.0
```

in group 1 at $t = 6$ (34.0%). Therefore, the McNemar test is useless in this particular situation. However, just as an example, the result of the McNemar test is presented in Output 6.2.

Output 6.2. Result of the McNemar test analysing the development over time of a dichotomous outcome variable Y_{dich} between $t = 1$ and $t = 6$

```
McNemar Test
      YDICHT1 OUTCOME VARIABLE Y AT T1 (2 GROUPS)
with YDICHT6 OUTCOME VARIABLE Y AT T6 (2 GROUPS)

                     YDICHT6
                 1.00      0.00        Cases            147
          0.00    17        80         Chi-Square    0.0000
YDICHT1
          1.00    32        18         Significance  1.0000
```

As expected, the McNemar test statistic chi-square $= 0.0000$ and the corresponding p-value is 1.0000, which indicates that there is no change over time for outcome variable Y_{dich}. Both outputs discussed so far illustrate perfectly the limitation of these two methods, i.e. only the difference between the changes over time in opposite directions is taken into account.

From the 2 × 2 table, also the total 'proportion of change' and the corresponding 95% confidence interval can be calculated. The 'proportion of change' is $(18 + 17)/147 = 0.24$. The standard error of this proportion, which is calculated according to Equation (6.3), is 0.035. With these two components the 95% confidence interval can be calculated, which leads to an interval that ranges from 0.17 to 0.31, indicating a highly significant change over time.

When the development over time of the outcome variable Y_{dich} is analysed using all six measurements, the multivariate extension of the McNemar test (Cochran's Q) can be used. However, Cochran's Q has the same limitations as the McNemar test. So again it is useless in this particular situation, in which the groups are defined according to the same (fixed) percentile at each measurement. However, Output 6.3 shows the result of the Cochran's Q test. As expected, the significance level of Cochran's Q (0.9945) is close to one, indicating no difference between the changes over time in opposite directions.

Output 6.3. Result of the Cochran's Q test calculated for the longitudinal development of the dichotomized outcome variable Y_{dich} from $t = 1$ to $t = 6$, using data from all repeated measurements

```
Cochran Q Test
Cases
        =0.00  =1.00  Variable
           97     50   YDICHT1   OUTCOME VARIABLE Y AT T1 (2 GROUPS)
           99     48   YDICHT2   OUTCOME VARIABLE Y AT T2 (2 GROUPS)
           96     51   YDICHT3   OUTCOME VARIABLE Y AT T3 (2 GROUPS)
           98     49   YDICHT4   OUTCOME VARIABLE Y AT T4 (2 GROUPS)
           99     48   YDICHT5   OUTCOME VARIABLE Y AT T5 (2 GROUPS)
           98     49   YDICHT6   OUTCOME VARIABLE Y AT T6 (2 GROUPS)

   Cases              Cochran Q      DF      Significance
    147                0.4298         5         0.9945
```

To evaluate the total change over time, Equation (6.6) can be used. First of all, the $(T - 1)$ 2×2 tables must be constructed (Output 6.4). From these tables, the total 'proportion of change' can be calculated.

The sum of the changes is 143, so the 'proportion of change' is $143/(147 \times 5) = 0.19$. The corresponding 95% confidence interval (based on the standard error calculated with Equation (6.3)) is [0.16 to 0.22], indicating a highly significant change over time.

Output 6.4. Five 2 x 2 tables used to calculate the 'proportion of change' when there are more than two measurements

		YDICHT2					YDICHT3		
	Count					Count			
				Row					Row
		0.00	1.00	Total			0.00	1.00	Total
YDICHT1					YDICHT2				
	0.00	83	14	97		0.00	83	16	99
	1.00	16	34	50		1.00	13	35	48
	Column	99	48	147		Column	96	51	147
		YDICHT4					YDICHT5		
	Count					Count			
				Row					Row
		0.00	1.00	Total			0.00	1.00	Total
YDICHT3					YDICHT4				
	0.00	84	12	96		0.00	86	12	98
	1.00	14	37	51		1.00	13	36	49
	Column	98	49	147		Column	99	48	147
		YDICHT6							
	Count								
				Row					
		0.00	1.00	Total					
YDICHT5									
	0.00	82	17	99					
	1.00	16	32	48					
	Column	98	49	147					

6.1.4.3 Comparing groups

When the aim of the study is to investigate whether there is a difference in development over time between several groups, the 'proportion of change' in the groups can be compared. In the example dataset the population can be divided into two groups, according to the time-independent predictor variable X_4 (i.e. males and females). For both groups a 2×2 table is constructed (Output 6.5), indicating the changes between $t = 1$ and $t = 6$ in Y_{dich}.

The next step is to calculate the 'proportion of change' for both groups. For the group $X_4 = 1$, $p_{\text{change}} = 13/69 = 0.19$; while for the group $X_4 = 2$, $p_{\text{change}} = 0.28$. From these two proportions the difference and the 95% confidence interval can be calculated. The latter is based on the standard

Output 6.5. 2 x 2 tables indicating the relationship between the outcome variable Y_{dich} at $t = 1$ and $t = 6$ for two groups divided by X_4 (i.e. gender)

```
X4 equals 1
YDICHT1 OUTCOME VARIABLE Y AT T1 (2 GROUPS)
by YDICHT6 OUTCOME VARIABLE Y AT T6 (2 GROUPS)
                        YDICHT1
                Count
                                          Row
                        0.00      1.00    Total
YDICHT6
                0.00    40          5      45
                                           65.2
                1.00     8         16      24
                                           34.8
                Column  48         21      69
                Total   69.6      30.4    100.0


X4 equals 2
YDICHT1 OUTCOME VARIABLE Y AT T1 (2 GROUPS)
by YDICHT6 OUTCOME VARIABLE Y AT T6 (2 GROUPS)
                        YDICHT6
                Count
                                          Row
                        0.00      1.00    Total
YDICHT1
                0.00    40         12      52
                                           66.7
                1.00    10         16      26
                                           33.3
                Column  50         28      78
                        64.1      35.9    100.0
```

error calculated with Equation (6.5). The difference in 'proportion of change' between the two groups is 0.09, with a 95% confidence interval of $[-0.05$ to 0.23]. So, there is a difference between the two groups (i.e. females have a 9% greater change over time), but this difference is not statistically significant.

When there are more than two measurements, Equation (6.4) can be used to calculate the 'proportion of change' in both groups. After creating $(T - 1)$ separate 2×2 tables, for group $X_4 = 1$ this proportion equals 0.18, and for group $X_4 = 2$, this proportion equals 0.21. The difference in 'proportion of change' between the two groups (i.e. 0.03) can be tested for significance by means of the 95% confidence interval. Based on the standard error, which is calculated with Equation (6.5), this interval is $[-0.03$ to $0.09]$, so the (small) difference observed between the two groups is not statistically significantly different from zero.

6.2 Relationships with other variables

6.2.1 'Traditional' methods

With the (simple) methods described in Section 6.1 it was possible to answer the question of whether there is a change/development over time in a certain dichotomous outcome variable, and whether there is a difference in change/development over time between two or more groups. Both questions can also be answered by using more complicated methods, which must be applied in any other situation than described above, for instance to answer the question of whether there is a relationship between the development of a dichotomous outcome variable Y_{dich} and one or more predictor variables X. In Section 4.2, it was discussed that for continuous outcome variables 'traditional', i.e. cross-sectional, methods are sometimes used to analyse these longitudinal relationships. For dichotomous outcome variables, comparable procedures are available. The most popular choice is the method illustrated in Figure 4.2, i.e. 'long-term exposure' to certain predictor variables is related to the dichotomous outcome variable at the end of the follow-up period. It is obvious that this analysis can be performed with (simple) cross-sectional logistic regression analysis.

6.2.2 Example

Output 6.6 presents the results of a logistic regression analysis, in which the 'long-term exposures' to the predictor variables X_1 to X_4 between $t = 1$ and $t = 6$ (using all available data) are related to the outcome variable Y_{dich} at $t = 6$.

From the significance levels it can be seen that 'long-term exposure' to X_2 is significantly associated with Y_{dich} at $t = 6$. The level of significance is based on the Wald statistic, which is defined as the regression coefficient divided

Output 6.6. Results of a logistic regression analysis relating 'long-term exposures' to predictor variables X_1 to X_4 between $t = 1$ and $t = 6$ (using all available data) to the dichotomous outcome variable Y_{dich} at $t = 6$

	B	Std. error	Wald	df	Sig
Constant	-5.863	2.873	4.165	1	0.000
X1	1.438	1.120	1.648	1	0.199
AveragX2	0.861	0.205	17.680	1	0.000
AveragX3	-0.122	0.391	0.097	1	0.755
X4	-0.607	0.500	1.472	1	0.225

Dependent variable: DICHOTOMOUS OUTCOME VARIABLE YDICH AT T6

by its standard error, squared. The Wald statistic follows a χ^2 distribution with (in this case) one degree of freedom. The corresponding odds ratio can be calculated as exp(regression coefficient), which is equal to 2.36, and the 95% confidence interval can be calculated as exp(regression coefficient ± 1.96 times the standard error of the regression coefficient), which is [1.58 to 3.53]. The interpretation of the odds ratio is straightforward: a one point difference in the 'long-term exposure' to X_2 between two subjects is associated with a 2.37 times higher odds of being in the upper tertile of the outcome variable Y_{dich} at $t = 6$. It should be noted that a 2.37 times higher odds is usually (loosely) interpreted as a 2.37 times greater 'risk', which is comparable but not the same.

6.2.3 Sophisticated methods

In general, when a dichotomous outcome variable is used in a longitudinal study, and the objective of the study is to analyse the relationship between the development of such a variable and the development of one or more predictor variables, it is possible to use the sophisticated methods mentioned before (i.e. GEE analysis and random coefficient analysis). In Chapter 4, it was extensively explained that for continuous outcome variables in longitudinal studies the sophisticated techniques can be considered as 'longitudinal linear regression analysis'. Analogous to this, GEE analysis and random coefficient analysis of a dichotomous outcome variable in longitudinal studies can be considered as 'longitudinal logistic regression analysis'. So, comparable to Equation (4.3), the longitudinal logistic model can be formulated as in Equation (6.6).

$$\ln\left(\frac{\Pr\left(Y_{it}=1\right)}{1-\Pr\left(Y_{it}=1\right)}\right) = \beta_0 + \sum_{j=1}^{j}\beta_{1j} + \beta_2 t + \sum_{k=1}^{K}\beta_{3k}Z_{ikt}$$

$$+ \sum_{m=1}^{M}\beta_{4m}G_{im} \tag{6.6a}$$

In a different notation:

$$\Pr(Y_{it}=1)$$

$$= \frac{1}{1+\exp\left[-\left(\beta_0 + \sum_{j=1}^{J}\beta_{1j}X_{itj} + \beta_2 t + \sum_{k=1}^{K}\beta_{3k}Z_{ikt} + \sum_{m=1}^{M}\beta_{4m}G_{im}\right)\right]}$$

$$\tag{6.6b}$$

where $\Pr(Y_{it}=1)$ is the probability that the observations at t_1 to t_T of subject i equal 1 (where T is the the number of measurements and 1 means that subject i belongs to the group of interest), β_0 is the intercept, X_{ijt} is the independent variable j of subject i at time t, β_{1j} is the regression coefficient of independent variable j, J is the number of independent variables, t is time, β_2 is the regression coefficient of time, Z_{ikt} is the time-dependent covariate k of subject i at time t, β_{3k} is the regression coefficient of time-dependent covariate k, K is the number of time-dependent covariates, G_{im} is the time-independent covariate m of subject i, β_{4m} is the regression coefficient of time-independent covariate m, and M is the number of time-independent covariates.

Although the model looks quite complicated, it is in fact nothing more than an extension of the (simple) logistic regression model. The extension is presented in the subscript t, which indicates that the same individuals can be repeatedly measured over time. In this model the probability of belonging to a group (coded 1) from t_1 to t_T (Y_{it}) is related to several predictor variables (X_{ijt}), several time-dependent covariates (Z_{ikt}), several time-independent covariates (G_{im}) and time (t). Like in (simple) multiple logistic regression analysis, all predictor variables and covariates can be continuous, dichotomous or categorical, although in the latter situation dummy coding can or must be used. The coefficient of interest is β_1, because this coefficient reflects the relationship between the development of a certain predictor variable (X_{it}) and belonging to the group of interest from t_1 to t_T. Like in simple logistic regression, this coefficient (β_1) can be transformed into an odds ratio ($\exp(\beta_1)$). The interpretation of the regression coefficients (i.e. odds ratios) is equivalent to the 'combined' interpretation of the regression coefficients for continuous outcome variables (see the example in Section 6.2.4 for a detailed explanation).

Analogous to the situation with continuous outcome variables, with GEE analysis a correction is made for the within-subject correlations between the repeated measurements by assuming a 'working correlation structure', while with random coefficient analysis this correction is made by allowing different regression coefficients to be random.

6.2.4 Example
6.2.4.1 Generalized estimating equations

For dichotomous outcome variables, the GEE approach also requires the choice of a 'working correlation structure'. Although there are the same possibilities as have been discussed for continuous outcome variables (see Section 4.5.2), it is not possible to use the correlation structure of the observed data as a guide for the choice of 'working correlation structure'. In this example, an exchangeable correlation structure (which is the default option in many software packages) will be used.

Output 6.7 presents the result of the logistic GEE analysis in which Y_{dich} is related to the four predictor variables (X_1 to X_4), and time.

The output of the so-called binomial generalized estimating equations is comparable to the output of a linear GEE analysis, which was discussed in Section 4.5.4.2. The outcome variable is YDICH, which is the dichotomized version of the outcome variable Y, and the correlation structure used is 'exchangeable'. The second part of the output consists of the parameter estimates. For each of the predictor variables the magnitude of the regression coefficients, the standard error and the corresponding p-values are presented. In addition, for the logistic GEE analysis, the odds ratio and the corresponding 95% confidence intervals are also shown. With regard to the four predictor variables, only X_2 is significantly related to the development of

Output 6.7. Results of the logistic GEE analysis performed on the example dataset

```
Binomial Generalized Estimating Equations
Response: YDICH   Corr: Exchangeable
Column   Name        Coeff   StErr   p-value   Odds    95%      CI
-----------------------------------------------------------------------
     0   Constant   -2.270   1.916   0.236
     2   TIME       -0.077   0.037   0.039    0.926   0.861    0.996
     4   X1          0.222   0.757   0.770    1.248   0.283    5.507
     5   X2          0.340   0.063   0.000    1.404   1.242    1.588
     6   X3         -0.151   0.198   0.446    0.860   0.583    1.267
     7   X4          0.084   0.374   0.822    1.088   0.523    2.264
-----------------------------------------------------------------------
n:147   s:0.982   #iter:13
Estimate of common correlation 0.488
```

the dichotomous outcome variable Y_{dich}. The regression coefficient is 0.340, and the odds ratio is 1.404. The 95% confidence interval ranges from 1.242 to 1.588. The interpretation of this odds ratio is somewhat complicated. As for the regression coefficients calculated for a continuous outcome variable, the odds ratios can be interpreted in two ways. (1) The 'cross-sectional' or 'between-subjects' interpretation: a subject with a one-unit higher score for predictor variable X_2, compared to another subject, has a 1.404 times higher odds of being in the highest group for the dichotomous outcome variable Y_{dich}. (2) The 'longitudinal' or 'within-subject' interpretation: an increase of one unit in predictor variable X_2 within a subject over a certain time period is associated with a 1.404 times higher odds of moving to the highest group of the dichotomous outcome variable Y_{dich} compared to the situation in which no change occurs in predictor variable X_2. The magnitude of the regression coefficient (i.e. the magnitude of the odds ratio) reflects both relationships, and it is not clear from the results of this analysis which is the most important component of the relationship. In Section 6.2.6 an alternative model (i.e. an autoregressive model) will be presented, in which the 'longitudinal' part of the relationship can be more or less disconnected from the 'cross-sectional' part.

The last part of the output shows some additional information provided by the logistic GEE analysis: the number of subjects used in the analysis ($n = 147$), the scale parameter ($s = 0.982$), the number of iterations needed to create the result (#iter:13), and the estimate of common correlation (0.488). Because an exchangeable correlation structure was chosen, only one correlation coefficient is estimated.

As in the GEE analysis with a continuous outcome variable, the scale parameter (also known as dispersion parameter) is an indication of the variance of the model. The interpretation of this coefficient is, however, different to that in the situation with a continuous outcome variable. This has to do with the characteristics of the binomial distribution on which the logistic GEE analysis is based. In the binomial distribution the variance is directly linked to the mean value (Equation (6.7)).

$$\mathrm{var}(\bar{p}) = \bar{p}\,(1 - \bar{p}) \tag{6.7}$$

where var is the variance, and $\bar{p}$ is the the average probability.

So, for the logistic GEE analysis, the scale parameter has to be one (i.e. a direct connection between the variance and the mean). From Output 6.7, however, it can be seen that the scale parameter was slightly lower than one. It should be noted that in some software packages the scale parameter for the logistic GEE analysis is set at a fixed value of one (see Chapter 12).

It is somewhat surprising that time is significantly related to the development of outcome variable Y_{dich} (odds ratio of 0.926), because Y_{dich} is based on fixed cut-off points (i.e. tertiles), and there is only a small change (maximal 1%) over time. The reason for this negative relationship with time is the fact that multiple analysis is applied, i.e. a 'correction' is made for the four predictor variables. When a univariate GEE analysis is carried out, with only time as a predictor variable, the relationship is, as expected, far from significant (see Output 6.8).

Output 6.8. Results of the GEE analysis with only time as a predictor variable

```
Binomial Generalized Estimating Equations
Response: YDICH   Corr: Exchangeable
Column  Name        Coeff  StErr  p-value  Odds    95%    CI
---------------------------------------------------------------
     0  Constant   -0.667  0.175   0.000
     2  TIME       -0.006  0.031   0.844  0.994  0.935  1.056
---------------------------------------------------------------
n:147  s:1.001  #iter:9
Estimate of common correlation 0.513
```

Output 6.9. Results of the GEE analyses with an independent (A), a 5-dependent (B), and an unstructured correlation structure (C)

```
(A)Binomial Generalized Estimating Equations
Response: YDICH   Corr: Independence
Column  Name       Coeff  StErr  p-value  Odds   95%     CI
-------------------------------------------------------------
    0   Constant  -3.261  1.992   0.102
    2   TIME      -0.106  0.041   0.009   0.899  0.830   0.974
    4   X1         0.557  0.784   0.478   1.745  0.375   8.118
    5   X2         0.467  0.090   0.000   1.595  1.338   1.901
    6   X3        -0.125  0.248   0.614   0.882  0.542   1.436
    7   X4         0.046  0.395   0.908   1.047  0.482   2.272
-------------------------------------------------------------
n:147   s:0.997   #iter:12
```

```
(B)Binomial Generalized Estimating Equations
Response: YDICH   Corr: 5-Dependence
Column  Name       Coeff  StErr  p-value  Odds   95%     CI
-------------------------------------------------------------
    0   Constant  -2.259  1.915   0.238
    2   TIME      -0.073  0.038   0.052   0.929  0.863   1.001
    4   X1         0.228  0.758   0.763   1.257  0.285   5.549
    5   X2         0.331  0.061   0.000   1.392  1.235   1.569
    6   X3        -0.129  0.193   0.504   0.879  0.602   1.283
    7   X4         0.083  0.373   0.824   1.087  0.523   2.258
-------------------------------------------------------------
n:147   s:0.98   #iter:13
Estimate of common correlations 0.549, 0.517, 0.453, 0.486, 0.479
```

```
(C)Binomial Generalized Estimating Equations
Response: YDICH   Corr: Unspecified
Column  Name       Coeff  StErr  p-value  Odds   95%     CI
-------------------------------------------------------------
    0   Constant  -2.194  1.904   0.249
    2   TIME      -0.077  0.036   0.035   0.926  0.862   0.995
    4   X1         0.225  0.756   0.766   1.253  0.284   5.518
    5   X2         0.321  0.057   0.000   1.379  1.233   1.542
    6   X3        -0.110  0.188   0.560   0.896  0.619   1.296
    7   X4         0.082  0.370   0.824   1.086  0.526   2.242
-------------------------------------------------------------
n:147   s:0.978   #iter:13
Estimate of common correlation
1.000   0.565   0.466   0.395   0.491   0.446
0.565   1.000   0.536   0.616   0.532   0.445
0.466   0.536   1.000   0.552   0.553   0.392
0.395   0.616   0.552   1.000   0.559   0.375
0.491   0.532   0.553   0.559   1.000   0.462
0.446   0.445   0.392   0.375   0.462   1.000
```

Table 6.1. Results of the GEE analysis with different correlation structures

| | Correlation structure | | | |
	Independent	Exchangeable	5-Dependent	Unstructured
X_1	0.56 (0.78)	0.22 (0.76)	0.23 (0.76)	0.23 (0.76)
X_2	0.47 (0.09)	0.34 (0.06)	0.33 (0.06)	0.32 (0.06)
X_3	−0.13 (0.25)	−0.15 (0.20)	−0.13 (0.19)	−0.11 (0.19)
X_4	0.05 (0.40)	0.08 (0.37)	0.08 (0.37)	0.08 (0.37)
Time	−0.11 (0.04)	−0.08 (0.04)	−0.07 (0.04)	−0.08 (0.04)

The results presented in Output 6.8 also indicate that a GEE analysis regarding the longitudinal relationship with time has the same disadvantages as have been mentioned for the McNemar test and Cochran's Q. So, on average there is no change over time in the dichotomous outcome variable Y_{dich}.

Comparable to the situation already described for continuous outcome variables, GEE analysis requires the choice of a particular 'working correlation structure'. It has already been mentioned that for a dichotomous outcome variable it is not possible to base that choice on the correlation structure of the observed data. It is therefore interesting to investigate the difference in regression coefficients estimated when different correlation structures are chosen. Output 6.9 shows the results of several analyses with different correlation structures and Table 6.1 summarizes the results of the different GEE analyses.

The most important conclusion which can be drawn from Table 6.1 is that the results of the GEE analysis with different correlation structures are highly comparable. This finding is different from that observed in the analysis of a continuous outcome variable (see Table 4.2), for which a remarkable difference was found between the results of the analysis with different correlation structures. So, (probably) the statement in the literature that GEE analysis is robust against the wrong choice of a correlation structure is particularly true for dichotomous outcome variables (see for instance also Liang and Zeger, 1993).

Furthermore, from Table 6.1 it can be seen that there are remarkable differences between the results obtained from the analysis with an **independent** correlation structure and the results obtained from the analysis with the three **dependent** correlation structures. It should further be noted that the standard errors obtained from the analysis with an independent correlation structure are higher than those obtained from the analysis with a dependent correlation structure. This 'over-estimation' is irrespective of the nature of the particular predictor variable. Although the over-estimation is more pronounced for the time-dependent predictor variables, it should be noted that this differs from the situation with a continuous outcome variable.

To put the results of the GEE analysis in a somewhat broader perspective, they can be compared with the results of a 'naive' logistic regression analysis, in which the dependency of observations is ignored. Output 6.10 presents the results of such a 'naive' logistic regression analysis.

Output 6.10. Results of a 'naive' logistic regression analysis performed on the example dataset, ignoring the dependency of the observations

```
Logistic Regression Analysis
Response: YDICH
Column  Name       Coeff   StErr  p-value   Odds    95%      CI
-----------------------------------------------------------------
     0  Constant  -3.261   1.077   0.002
     2  TIME      -0.106   0.047   0.024   0.899   0.820   0.986
     4  X1         0.557   0.434   0.199   1.745   0.746   4.083
     5  X2         0.467   0.061   0.000   1.595   1.415   1.798
     6  X3        -0.125   0.209   0.550   0.882   0.585   1.330
     7  X4         0.046   0.191   0.811   1.047   0.719   1.523
-----------------------------------------------------------------
df:876   Dev:1044.508   %(0):66.553   #iter:11   RSq: 0.071
```

The comparison between the results of the 'naive' logistic regression and the results of the GEE analysis with an independent correlation structure is different to what has been observed for continuous outcome variables. The regression coefficients are exactly the same as the regression coefficients obtained from a GEE analysis, while the standard errors obtained from the GEE analysis are higher than those calculated with the 'naive' logistic regression analysis, irrespective of the nature of the predictor variables. The only exception, however, is the standard error of time.

6.2.4.2 *Random coefficient analysis*

Comparable to the situation with continuous outcome variables, in the case of dichotomous outcome variables it is also possible to analyse the relationship with several predictor variables by means of random coefficient analysis. The first step is to perform an analysis with only a random intercept. Output 6.11 shows the result of this analysis.

Output 6.11. Results of a random coefficient analysis with only a random intercept

```
Random-effects logit                          Number of obs      =      882
Group variable (i) : id                       Number of groups   =      147
Random effects u_i ~ Gaussian                 Obs per group: min =        6
                                                             avg =      6.0
                                                             max =        6

                                              Wald chi2(5)       =    30.39
Log likelihood = -400.59729                   Prob > chi2        =   0.0000
```

ydich	Coeff	Std. Err.	z	P > |z|	[95% Conf. Interval]	
x1	0.8828525	1.81259	0.487	0.626	-2.669758	4.435463
x2	0.6991612	0.1442835	4.846	0.000	0.4163708	0.9819517
x3	-0.2489498	0.3615913	-0.688	0.491	-0.9576558	0.4597561
x4	0.3350076	0.713474	0.470	0.639	-1.063376	1.733391
time	-0.1552925	0.0718681	-2.161	0.031	-0.2961514	-0.0144335
_cons	-5.772749	4.327476	-1.334	0.182	-14.25445	2.708948
/lnsig2u	1.813016	0.193079	9.390	0.000	1.434588	2.191444
sigma_u	2.475662	0.2389992			2.048882	2.991341
rho	0.859726	0.0232848			0.8076152	0.8994785

```
Likelihood ratio test of rho=0:  chi2(1) = 243.31  Prob > chi2 = 0.0000
```

The output of a random coefficient analysis with a dichotomous outcome variable is comparable to the output observed for a continuous outcome variable.

The first part provides some general information about the model. It shows that a logistic random coefficient analysis was performed (random-effects logit) and that the random coefficients are normally distributed (random effects u_i ~ Gaussian). Furthermore, the log likelihood of the model and the result of a Wald test (Wald chi2(5) = 30.39), and the corresponding p-value (prob > chi2 = 0.000) are presented. This Wald test is a generalized Wald test for **all** predictor variables. Because X_1, X_2, X_3, X_4 and time are analysed in the model, the generalized Wald statistic follows a χ^2 distribution with five degrees of freedom, which is highly significant.

The second part of the output shows the most important information obtained from the analysis, i.e. the (fixed) regression coefficients. This information is exactly the same as has been discussed for continuous outcome variables, although the regression coefficients can be transformed into odds ratios by taking exp(coef). Again the interpretation of the coefficients is the same as has been discussed for the GEE analysis with dichotomous outcome variables, i.e. a combined 'between-subjects' (cross-sectional) and 'within-subject' (longitudinal) interpretation. For instance, for predictor variable X_2 the 'between-subjects' interpretation is that a subject with a one-unit higher score for predictor variable X_2, compared to another subject, has an exp(0.699) = 2.01 times higher odds of being in the highest group for the dichotomous outcome variable Y_{dich}. The 'within-subject' interpretation is that an increase of one unit in predictor variable X_2 within a subject (over a certain time period) is associated with a 2.01 times higher odds of moving to the highest group of the dichotomous outcome variable Y_{dich}, compared to the situation in which no change occurs in predictor variable X_2.

The last part of the output shows information about the random part of the analysis. The variance of the (normally distributed) random intercepts is denoted as sigma_u, and rho is an estimate of the within-subject correlation. Although it is of little interest, the output of the random coefficient analysis also shows the natural log of sigma_u (lnsig2u).

The likelihood ratio test of rho = 0 provides information on the importance of allowing a random intercept. The result of the likelihood ratio test presented here is based on the comparison between this model and a similar model without a random intercept. Apparently, this difference is 243.31, which follows a χ^2 distribution with one degree of freedom (i.e. the random intercept), and which is highly significant. In other words, the results of the likelihood ratio test suggest that it is necessary to allow a random intercept in this particular situation.

To verify the results of the likelihood ratio test, Output 6.12 presents the results of an analysis with no random intercept.

Output 6.12. Results of a random coefficient analysis with no random intercept

Logit estimates				Number of obs	=	882
				LR chi2(5)	=	79.68
				Prob > chi2	=	0.0000
Log likelihood = -522.25411				Pseudo R2	=	0.0709

ydich	Odds Ratio	Std. Err.	z	P > |z|	[95% Conf. Interval]	
x1	1.745148	0.7570111	1.284	0.199	0.7457575	4.083823
x2	1.594749	0.0974273	7.639	0.000	1.414784	1.797606
x3	0.8824154	0.1847934	-0.597	0.550	0.585351	1.330239
x4	1.04677	0.2004081	0.239	0.811	0.7192596	1.523411
time	0.8990267	0.0423753	-2.258	0.024	0.8196936	0.9860379

For this particular purpose, the only important information is the log likelihood of the model analysed (-522.25411). The difference between this value and the log likelihood of a model **with** a random intercept is 121.65682. The difference between the -2 log likelihoods is therefore 243.31, i.e. exactly the same as has been seen in Output 6.11.

So, from comparison of the -2 log likelihoods of the two models it can be concluded that allowing a random intercept is important. The next step is to evaluate the necessity of a random slope with time. Therefore a random coefficient analysis is performed, with both a random intercept and a random slope with time (Output 6.13).

To evaluate the necessity of a random slope with time, the log likelihood of the model presented in Output 6.13 (-397.84608) is compared to the log likelihood of the model with only a random intercept (-400.59729, Output 6.11). The difference between the two values is 2.75121. Two times this difference follows a χ^2 distribution with **two** degrees of freedom (i.e. the random slope and the covariance/correlation between the random slope and the random intercept), which gives a p-value of 0.064. This is not significant, so following the basic rule of significance, allowing a random slope with time is not really necessary. However, although the corresponding p-value is not significant, the difference in -2 log likelihood is substantial, so in this situation it is recommended to use a model with both a random intercept and a random slope with time.

Output 6.13. Results of a random coefficient analysis with a random intercept and a random slope with time

```
log likelihood = -397.84608
-------------------------------------------------------------------------
ydich      Coeff     Std. Err.      z      P > |z|     [95% Conf. Interval]
-------------------------------------------------------------------------
  x1      0.3276885   1.633606    0.201     0.841    -2.874121    3.529498
  x2      0.7158125   0.1373508   5.212     0.000     0.4466099   0.9850152
  x3     -0.22697     0.3574447  -0.635     0.525    -0.9275488   0.4736088
  x4      0.4606241   0.6981993   0.660     0.509    -0.9078214   1.82907
 time    -0.0685773   0.0952798  -0.720     0.472    -0.2553222   0.1181676
_cons    -5.304992    3.890947   -1.363     0.173    -12.93111    2.321123
-------------------------------------------------------------------------

Variances and covariances of random effects
-------------------------------------------------------------------------
  ***level 2 (id)
  var(1): 13.116573    (4.3382583)
cov(1,2): -1.0355152   (0.61205904)    cor(1,2): -0.8643663
  var(2):  0.10942006  (0.09086733)
```

6.2.5 Comparison between GEE analysis and random coefficient analysis

For continuous outcome variables it was seen that GEE analysis and random coefficient analysis provided almost identical results in the analysis of a longitudinal dataset. For dichotomous outcome variables, however, the situation is more complex. In Table 6.2 the results of the GEE analysis and the random coefficient analysis with a dichotomous outcome variable are summarized.

From Table 6.2 it can be concluded that there are remarkable differences between the results of the GEE analysis and the results of the random coefficient analysis. All regression coefficients and standard errors obtained from GEE analysis are much lower than those obtained from random coefficient analysis (except the regression coefficient for time when both a random intercept and a random slope with time are considered).

In this respect, it is important to realize that the regression coefficients calculated with GEE analysis are 'population averaged', i.e. the average of

Table 6.2. Regression coefficients and standard errors (in parentheses) of longitudinal regression analyses with a dichotomous outcome variable; a comparison between GEE analysis and random coefficient analysis

	GEE analysis[a]	Random coefficient analysis[b]	Random coefficient analysis[c]
X_1	0.22 (0.76)	0.88 (1.81)	0.33 (1.63)
X_2	0.34 (0.06)	0.70 (0.14)	0.72 (0.14)
X_3	−0.15 (0.20)	−0.25 (0.36)	−0.23 (0.36)
X_4	0.08 (0.37)	0.34 (0.71)	0.46 (0.70)
Time	−0.08 (0.04)	−0.16 (0.07)	−0.07 (0.10)

[a] GEE analysis with an exchangeable correlation structure.
[b] Random coefficient analysis with only a random intercept.
[c] Random coefficient analysis with a random intercept and a random slope with time.

the individual regression lines. The regression coefficients calculated with random coefficient analysis can be seen as 'subject specific'. In Figure 6.1, this difference is illustrated for both the linear model (i.e. with a continuous outcome variable) and the logistic model (i.e. with a dichotomous outcome variable) with only a random intercept. For the linear longitudinal regression analysis, both GEE analysis and random coefficient analysis produce exactly the same results, i.e. the 'population-average' is equal to the 'subject-specific' (see also Section 4.7). For the logistic longitudinal regression analysis, however, the two approaches produce different results. This has to do with the fact that in logistic regression analysis the intercept has a different interpretation than in linear regression analysis. From Figure 6.1 it can be seen that the regression coefficients calculated with a logistic GEE analysis will always be lower than the coefficients calculated with a logistic random coefficient analysis (see for instance also Neuhaus et al., 1991; Hu et al., 1998). It should further be noted that when a random coefficient analysis is performed with time as the only predictor variable, no significant change over time is detected in outcome variable Y_{dich} (results not shown in detail). In other words, despite the fact that random coefficient analysis is a 'subject-specific' approach, the analysis of the development of a dichotomous outcome variable over time has the same disadvantages as has been mentioned for GEE analysis.

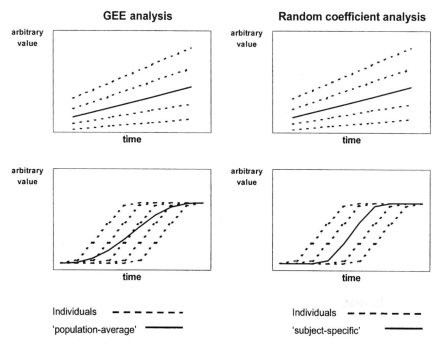

Figure 6.1. Illustration of the 'population average' approach of GEE analysis and the 'subject specific' approach of random coefficient analysis, illustrating both the situation with a continuous outcome variable (upper graphs) and the situation with a dichotomous outcome variable (lower graphs).

Because of the remarkable differences, the question then arises: 'When a dichotomous outcome variable is analysed in a longitudinal study, should GEE analysis or random coefficient analysis be used?' If one is performing a population study and one is interested in the relationship between a dichotomous outcome variable and several other predictor variables, GEE analysis will probably provide the most 'valid' results. However, if one is interested in the individual development over time of a dichotomous outcome variable, random coefficient analysis will probably provide the most 'valid' results. It should, however, also be noted that random coefficient analyses with a dichotomous outcome variable have not yet been fully developed. Different software packages give different results, and within one software package there is (usually) more than one algorithm to estimate the coefficients. Unfortunately, these different estimation procedures often lead to different results (see also Chapter 12). In other words, although in theory random coefficient

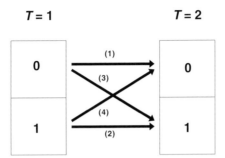

Figure 6.2. Changes in a dichotomous variable between two time-points lead to a categorical variable with four groups.

analysis is highly suitable in some situations, in practice one should be very careful in using this technique in the longitudinal analysis of a dichotomous outcome variable.

6.2.6 Alternative models

In Chapter 5 several alternative methods were introduced to analyse longitudinal relationships for continuous outcome variables (i.e. a time-lag model, the modelling of changes, and an autoregressive model). In principle, all the alternative models discussed for continuous outcome variables can also be used for the analysis of dichotomous outcome variables. The time-lag model can be used when one is interested in the analysis of possible causation, while an autoregressive model can be used when one is interested in the analysis of the 'longitudinal' part of the relationship. However, a problem arises in the modelling of changes between subsequent measurements. This has to do with the fact that changes in a dichotomous outcome variable result in a categorical variable with four groups (i.e. subjects who stay in one group, subjects who stay in another group and two groups in which subjects move from one group to another (see Figure 6.2)), and with the fact that the longitudinal analysis of categorical outcome variables is rather complicated (see Chapter 7).

This chapter does not include a very detailed discussion of the results of alternative models to analyse dichotomous outcome variables, because this was already done in Chapter 5 with regard to continuous outcome variables. Basically, the same problems and advantages apply to dichotomous outcome variables. It is important to realize that the three models represent different aspects of the longitudinal relationships between a dichotomous outcome variable and several predictor variables, and that therefore the regression coefficients obtained from the different models should be interpreted differently.

6.2.7 Comments

In this chapter, the longitudinal analysis of a dichotomous outcome variable is explained in a rather simple way. It should be realized that the technical details of these analyses are very complicated. For these technical details reference should be made to other publications (with regard to GEE analysis for instance Liang and Zeger, 1986; Prentice, 1988; Lipsitz et al., 1991; Carey et al., 1993; Diggle et al., 1994; Lipsitz et al., 1994b; Wiliamson et al., 1995; Lipsitz and Fitzmaurice, 1996; and with regard to random coefficient analysis for instance Conway, 1990; Goldstein, 1995; Rodriguez and Goldman, 1995; Goldstein and Rasbash, 1996; Gibbons and Hedeker, 1997; Barbosa and Goldstein, 2000; Yang and Goldstein, 2000; Rodriguez and Goldman, 2001).

Categorical and 'count' outcome variables

7.1 Categorical outcome variables

7.1.1 Two measurements

Longitudinal analysis with a categorical outcome variable is more problematic than the longitudinal analysis of continuous or dichotomous outcome variables. Until recently only simple methods were available to analyse such outcome variables. Therefore, categorical variables are sometimes treated as continuous, especially when they are ordinal and have a sufficient number (usually five or more) of categories. Another method is to reduce the categorical outcome variable into a dichotomous one by combining two or more categories. However, this results in a loss of information, and is only recommended when there are only a few subjects in one or more categories of the categorical variable.

The simplest form of longitudinal study with a categorical outcome variable is one where the categorical outcome variable is measured twice in time. This situation (when the categorical variable consists of three groups) is illustrated in the 3×3 table presented below (where n stands for number of subjects and p stands for proportion of the total number of subjects N).

		t_2			
		1	2	3	Total
t_1	1	$n_{11}(p_{11})$	$n_{12}(p_{12})$	$n_{13}(p_{13})$	$n_{1(t1)}(p_{1(t1)})$
	2	$n_{21}(p_{21})$	$n_{22}(p_{22})$	$n_{13}(p_{13})$	$n_{2(t1)}(p_{2(t1)})$
	3	$n_{31}(p_{31})$	$n_{32}(p_{32})$	$n_{33}(p_{33})$	$n_{3(t1)}(p_{3(t1)})$
	Total	$n_{1(t2)}(p_{1(t2)})$	$n_{2(t2)}(p_{2(t2)})$	$n_{3(t2)}(p_{3(t2)})$	$N(1)$

To determine whether there is a development or change over time in the categorical outcome variable Y_{cat}, an extension of the McNemar test (which has been discussed for dichotomous outcome variables, see Section 6.1.1) can be used. This extension is known as the Stuart–Maxwell statistic, and is only suitable for outcome variables with three categories. The Stuart–Maxwell statistic follows a χ^2 distribution with one degree of freedom, and is defined as shown in Equation (7.1).

$$\chi^2 = \frac{\overline{n_{23}}d_1^2 + \overline{n_{13}}d_2^2 + \overline{n_{12}}d_3^2}{2(\overline{n_{12}}\,\overline{n_{13}} + \overline{n_{12}}\,\overline{n_{23}} + \overline{n_{13}}\,\overline{n_{23}})} \tag{7.1a}$$

$$\overline{n_{ij}} = \frac{n_{ij} + n_{ji}}{2} \tag{7.1b}$$

$$d_i = n_{it1} - n_{it2} \tag{7.1c}$$

where n_{ij} is the number of subjects in group i at $t = 1$ and in group j at $t = 2$, and n_{ji} is the number of subjects in group j at $t = 1$ and in group i at $t = 2$.

Just as the McNemar test, the Stuart–Maxwell statistic gives an indication of the differences between the changes over time in opposite directions, while the main interest is usually the total change over time. Therefore, the 'proportion of change' can be calculated. This 'proportion of change' is a summation of all the off-diagonal proportions of the categorical 3×3 table, which is equal to $1 - (p_{11} + p_{22} + p_{33})$. Around this proportion a 95% confidence interval can be calculated in the usual way (for calculation of the standard error of the 'proportion of change', Equation (6.3) can be used). In addition to giving an indication of the precision of the 'proportion of change', this 95% confidence interval provides an answer to the question of whether there is a significant change over time. As for the dichotomous outcome variables, this procedure can be carried out for the proportion of subjects that 'increases' over time or the proportion of subjects that 'decreases' over time. It is obvious that the calculation of the 'proportion of change' is not limited to categorical variables with only three measurements.

7.1.2 More than two measurements

When there are more than two measurements in a longitudinal study, the same procedure can be followed as has been described for dichotomous outcome variables, i.e. the 'proportion of change' can be used as a measure of total change over time. To do so, $(T-1)\, r \times c$ tables[1] must be constructed (for $t=1$ and $t=2$, for $t=2$ and $t=3$, and so on), then for each table the 'proportion of change' can be calculated. To obtain the total 'proportion of change', Equation (7.2) can be applied:

$$\bar{p} = \frac{1}{N(T-1)} \sum_{i=1}^{N} c_i \tag{7.2}$$

where $\bar{p}$ is the overall 'proportion of change', N is the number of subjects, T is the number of measurements, and c_i is the number of changes for individual i.

7.1.3 Comparing groups

In research situations in which the longitudinal development over time between several groups must be compared, the simple methods discussed for dichotomous outcome variables can also be used for categorical outcome variables, i.e. comparing the 'proportion of change' between different groups, or comparing the 'proportion of change' in a certain direction between different groups. When there are only two groups to compare, a 95% confidence interval can be constructed around the difference in proportions, so that this difference can be tested for significance. This should be done in exactly the same way as has been described for dichotomous outcome variables (see Section 6.1.3).

7.1.4 Example

For the example, the original continuous outcome variable Y of the example dataset was divided into three equal groups, according to the 33rd and the 66th percentile, in order to create Y_{cat}. This was done at each of the six measurements (see also Section 1.4). Most of the statistical methods are suitable for situations in which there are only two measurements, and therefore the development between the first and the last repeated measurement (between $t=1$ and $t=6$) for the categorical outcome variable Y_{cat} will be considered first. In Output 7.1 the 3×3 table for Y_{cat} at $t=1$ and Y_{cat} at $t=6$ is presented. From Output 7.1 the Stuart–Maxwell statistic and the 'proportion of change' can be calculated. Unfortunately, the two indicators are not

---

[1] $r \times c$ stands for row $\times$ column, and indicates that all types of categorical variables can be analysed in this way.

Output 7.1. 3 x 3 table for the relationship between outcome variable Y_{cat} at $t = 1$ and Y_{cat} at $t = 6$

		YCATT6			Row
Count		1	2	3	Total
YCATT1					
	1	30	15	3	48
					32.7
	2	16	19	14	49
					33.3
	3	3	15	32	50
					34.0
	Column	49	49	49	147
	Total	33.3	33.3	33.3	100.0

Table 7.1. Two indicators for a change over time (between $t = 1$ and $t = 6$) for outcome variable Y_{cat}

Stuart–Maxwell statistic	$\chi^2 = 0.09$	$p = 0.76$
'proportion of change'	0.45	95% confidence interval 0.37–0.53

available in standard software packages, so they must be calculated manually. Table 7.1 shows the values of both indicators for a change over time.

With the Stuart–Maxwell statistic, the difference between the changes over time in opposite directions is tested for significance. Because the categorization of the outcome variable Y_{cat} was based on tertiles (i.e. fixed values), it is obvious that the Stuart–Maxwell statistic will be very low ($\chi^2 = 0.09$), and far from significant ($p = 0.76$). The 'proportion of change' is an indicator of the total change over time. The result indicates a 'moderate' and highly significant individual change over time.

When all the measurements are included in the analysis, the only possible way to investigate the individual change over time in a categorical outcome variable is to calculate the overall 'proportion of change'. To do so, all five 3×3 tables must be constructed. They are shown in Output 7.2. From the five 3×3 tables the total 'proportion of change' can be calculated (with Equation (7.2)). This proportion is equal to 0.35. The corresponding

Output 7.2. Five 3 x 3 tables to analyse the change over time in the outcome variable Y_{cat} between $t = 1$ and $t = 6$

		YCATT2 Count					YCATT3 Count		
		1	2	3			1	2	3
YCATT1					YCATT2				
	1	35	11	2		1	34	11	1
	2	8	29	12		2	18	20	15
	3	3	13	34		3	2	11	35

		YCATT4 Count					YCATT5 Count		
		1	2	3			1	2	3
YCATT3					YCATT4				
	1	45	9			1	36	16	
	2	7	23	12		2	10	24	12
	3		14	37		3	3	10	36

		YCATT6 Count		
		1	2	3
YCATT5				
	1	35	13	1
	2	12	22	16
	3	2	14	32

95% confidence interval (based on the standard error calculated with Equation (6.3)) is equal to [0.32 to 0.38], i.e. a highly significant change over time.

It is also possible to compare the development over time for outcome variable Y_{cat} between two or more groups. In the example, the development of Y_{cat} was compared between the two categories of time-independent predictor variable X_4 (i.e. gender). Output 7.3 shows the two 3 × 3 tables. For both groups the 'proportion of change' is exactly the same, i.e. 0.45. Around this (no) difference a 95% confidence interval can be constructed: [−0.16 to 0.16]. The width of the confidence interval provides information about the precision of the calculated difference between the two groups.

To obtain an estimation of the possible differences in development over time for the two groups by using all six measurements, the overall 'proportion

Output 7.3. 3 x 3 tables for the relationship between outcome variable Y_{cat} at t_1 and Y_{cat} at t_6 for the group in which X_4 equals 1 and for the group in which X_4 equals 2

```
X4 equals 1
YCATT1 OUTCOME VARIABLE Y AT T1 (3 GROUPS)
by YCATT6 OUTCOME VARIABLE Y AT T6 (3 GROUPS)
                      YCATT6
             Count
                                                    Row
                         1        2        3      Total
YCATT1
                1       14        7                  21
                                                   30.4
                2       11        8        5         24
                                                   34.8
                3        3        5       16         24
                                                   34.8
             Column     28       20       21         69
              Total    40.6     29.0     30.4      100.0
```

```
X4 equals 2
YCATT1 OUTCOME VARIABLE Y AT T1 (3 GROUPS)
by YCATT6 OUTCOME VARIABLE Y AT T6 (3 GROUPS)
                      YCATT6
             Count
                                                    Row
                         1        2        3      Total
YCATT1
                1       16        8        3         27
                                                   34.6
                2        5       11        9         25
                                                   32.1
                3               10       16         26
                                                   32.3
             Column     21       29       28         78
              Total    26.9     37.2     35.9      100.0
```

of change' must be calculated for both groups. When this is done (by creating $(T-1)$, 3 × 3 tables for both groups), the overall 'proportion of change' for the group X_4 equals 1 is 0.47, while for group X_4 equals 2, the overall proportion of change is 0.44. Around this difference of 3% a 95% confidence interval can be calculated. To obtain a standard error for this difference, Equation (6.5) can be applied to these data, which results in a confidence interval of $[-0.05$ to $0.11]$, i.e. no significant difference between the two groups.

7.1.5 Relationships with other variables

7.1.5.1 'Traditional' methods

With the (simple) methods described in the foregoing sections, it was possible to answer the question of whether there is a change/development over time in a certain categorical outcome variable and/or the question of whether there is a difference in change/development between two or more groups. Both questions can also be answered by using more complicated methods, which must be applied in any situation other than that described above: for instance, to answer the question of whether there is a relationship between the development of a categorical outcome variable Y_{cat} and one or more predictor variables X. For categorical outcome variables, a comparable 'cross-sectional' procedure is available, as has already been described for continuous and dichotomous outcome variables, i.e. 'long-term exposure' to certain predictor variables is related to the categorical outcome variable at the end of the follow-up period (see Figure 4.2). This analysis can be performed with polytomous logistic regression analysis, which is also known as multinomial logistic regression analysis, and is the categorical extension of logistic regression analysis.

7.1.5.2 Example

Output 7.4 presents the results of the polytomous logistic regression analysis, in which 'long-term exposures' to the predictor variables X_1 to X_4 between $t = 1$ and $t = 6$ (using all available data) were related to the categorical outcome variable Y_{cat} at $t = 6$.

With polytomous logistic regression analysis, basically two logistic regression analyses are combined into one analysis, although the procedure is slightly different from performing two separate independent logistic regression analyses. In the polytomous logistic regression analysis, the upper tertile of the outcome variable Y_{cat} is used as a reference category. The interpretation of the regression coefficients is exactly the same as for (simple) logistic regression analysis. From Output 7.4 it can be seen that, for instance,

Output 7.4. Results of a polytomous logistic regression analysis relating 'long-term exposures' to predictor variables X_1 to X_4 between $t=1$ and $t=6$ (using all available data) to the categorical outcome variable Y_{cat} at $t=6$

		B	Std. error	Wald	df	Sig
1	Constant	6.416	2.959	4.702	1	0.030
	X1	-1.213	1.299	0.872	1	0.350
	AveragX2	-1.036	0.257	16.191	1	0.000
	AveragX3	-0.177	0.455	0.151	1	0.697
	X4	0.527	0.580	0.824	1	0.364
2	Constant	6.695	2.852	5.511	1	0.019
	X1	-1.665	1.261	1.743	1	0.187
	AveragX2	-0.741	0.225	10.804	1	0.001
	AveragX3	0.359	0.435	1.623	1	0.203
	X4	0.714	0.560	1.623	1	0.203

Dependent variable: CATEGORICAL OUTCOME VARIABLE Y AT T6 (3 GROUPS)

'long-term exposure' to X_2 is significantly associated with the first group as well as the second group of the categorical outcome variable Y_{cat} at $t = 6$. The odds ratios for both groups can be obtained from the regression coefficients, i.e. the odds ratio is exp(regression coefficient) and the corresponding 95% confidence interval is exp(regression coefficient $\pm$ 1.96 times the standard error of the regression coefficient). The interpretation of the odds ratio is straightforward: a one-point difference in the 'long-term exposure' to X_2 between subjects is associated with a 0.35 (i.e. exp(-1.036)) 'higher' odds of being in the lowest tertile of the outcome variable Y_{cat} at $t = 6$, compared to the odds of being in the highest tertile, and a 0.48 (i.e. exp(-0.741)) 'higher' odds of being in the second tertile, compared to the odds of being in the highest tertile. The corresponding 95% confidence intervals are [0.21–0.59] and [0.31–0.74] respectively.

7.1.5.3 Sophisticated methods

In Chapters 4 and 6, it was argued that longitudinal data analysis with a continuous outcome variable is a longitudinal extension of linear regression analysis, and that longitudinal data analysis with a dichotomous outcome variable is a longitudinal extension of logistic regression analysis, i.e. both take into account the fact that the repeated measurements within one subject are correlated. Analogous to this, it is obvious that longitudinal data analysis with a categorical outcome variable is a longitudinal extension of polytomous logistic regression analysis. Polytomous logistic regression for longitudinal data analysis was first described for GEE analysis (see for instance Liang et al., 1992; Miller et al., 1993; Lipsitz et al., 1994b). Surprisingly this polytomous logistic GEE approach is still not yet available in standard software packages, and will therefore not be discussed in detail. The general idea of this GEE approach is the same as all other GEE approaches, i.e. a correction for the dependency of observations is performed by assuming a certain 'working correlation structure'.

In recent years, a polytomous logistic random coefficient analysis has also been described (Agresti et al., 2000; Rabe-Hesketh et al., 2001a; Rabe-Hesketh and Skondral, 2001). As with all other random coefficient analyses described earlier, with this newly developed method all questions can be answered that were answered by the earlier mentioned simple methods. Moreover, it can also be used to analyse the **longitudinal** relationship between a categorical outcome variable and one or more predictor variables. The underlying procedures and the interpretation of the regression coefficients are comparable to what has been described for logistic random coefficient analysis.

7.1.5.4 Example

The first step in the analysis to answer the question whether there is a relationship between the categorical outcome variable Y_{cat} and the four predictor variables (X_1 to X_4) and time is to perform a random coefficient analysis with only a random intercept. Output 7.5 shows the results of this analysis.

The structure of Output 7.5 is comparable to what has been seen for continuous and dichotomous outcome variables. First the log likelihood of the model analysed is presented (-784.6426), which is only interesting in comparison to the log likelihood value of another model, which must be an extension of the presented model. In the next part of the output, the regression coefficients and standard errors are given as well as the z-value (the regression coefficient divided by its standard error), the corresponding p-value and the 95% confidence intervals of the regression coefficients. In the example dataset, Y_{cat} is a categorical outcome variable with three categories (i.e. tertiles), so there are two 'tables' with regression coefficients. In the first 'table' the second tertile of Y_{cat} is compared to the lowest tertile of Y_{cat} (which is the reference category), while in the second 'table' the highest tertile of Y_{cat}

Output 7.5. Result of a random coefficient analysis with a categorical outcome variable and only a random intercept

```
log likelihood = -784.6426
------------------------------------------------------------------------
     ycat      Coeff      Std. Err.      z      P > |z|   [95% Conf.   Interval]
------------------------------------------------------------------------
c2
       x1   -0.8562861   1.513829    -0.566   0.572   -3.823336    2.110764
       x2    0.6193215   0.1712165    3.617   0.000    0.2837433   0.9548997
       x3   -0.0428614   0.3847279   -0.111   0.911   -0.7969143   0.7111915
       x4    0.1630424   0.6576949    0.248   0.804   -1.126016    1.452101
     time   -0.1380476   0.0753289   -1.833   0.067   -0.2856894   0.0095943
    _cons    0.4352662   3.829679     0.114   0.910   -7.070767    7.941299
------------------------------------------------------------------------
c3
       x1    0.0196611   1.520852     0.013   0.990   -2.961154    3.000476
       x2    0.9471408   0.1703437    5.560   0.000    0.6132733   1.281008
       x3   -0.3353352   0.3953064   -0.848   0.396   -1.110122    0.439451
       x4    0.281329    0.6609212    0.426   0.670   -1.014053    1.576711
     time   -0.2002512   0.0769589   -2.602   0.009   -0.3510879  -0.0494144
    _cons   -2.485896    3.846796    -0.646   0.518  -10.02548     5.053685
------------------------------------------------------------------------

Variances and covariances of random effects
------------------------------------------------------------------------
***level 2 (id)
var(1): 7.5624431 (1.6150762)
```

is compared to the lowest tertile. The interpretation of the regression coefficients is rather complicated. From Output 7.5 it can be seen that for instance X_2 is significantly related to the outcome variable Y_{cat}. For the comparison between the second tertile and the reference category (i.e. the lowest tertile) the regression coefficient (0.6193215) can be transformed into an odds ratio (i.e. $\exp(0.6193215) = 1.86$). As for all other longitudinal regression coefficients this odds ratio has a 'combined' interpretation. (1) The 'cross-sectional' or 'between-subjects' interpretation: a subject with a one-unit higher score for predictor variable X_2, compared to another subject, has a 1.86 times higher odds of being in the second tertile compared to the odds of being in the lowest tertile. (2) The 'longitudinal' or 'within-subject' interpretation: an increase of one unit in predictor variable X_2 within a subject (over a certain time period) is associated with a 1.86 times higher odds of moving from the lowest tertile to the second tertile of the categorical outcome variable Y_{cat}, compared to the situation in which no change occurs in predictor variable X_2. The regression coefficient of X_2 belonging to the comparison between the highest tertile and the lowest tertile ($\exp(0.9471408) = 2.58$) can be interpreted in the same way. (1) A subject with a one-unit higher score for predictor variable X_2, compared to another subject, has a 2.58 times higher odds of being in the highest tertile for the categorical outcome variable Y_{cat} compared to the odds of being in the lowest tertile. (2) The 'longitudinal' or 'within-subject' interpretation: an increase of one unit in predictor variable X_2 within a subject (over a certain time period) is associated with a 2.58 times higher odds of moving from the lowest tertile to the highest tertile of the categorical outcome variable Y_{cat}, compared to the situation in which no change occurs in predictor variable X_2. The magnitude of the regression coefficient (i.e. the magnitude of the odds ratio) reflects both relationships, and it is not clear from the results of this analysis, which is the most important component of the relationship. However, the relative contribution of both parts highly depends on the proportion of subjects who move from one category to another. In the example dataset for instance, the proportion of subjects who move from the lowest to the highest category is rather low, so for the comparison between the lowest and the highest tertile, the estimated odds ratio of 2.58 mainly reflects the 'between-subjects' relationship. As for all other longitudinal data analyses, alternative models are available (e.g. an autoregressive model, see Section 5.2.3) in which the 'between-subjects' and 'within-subject' relationships can be more or less separated.

In the last part of Output 7.5 the (normally distributed) random variation in intercept (7.5624431) with the corresponding standard error (1.6150762) is provided. Although the variation in intercepts between subjects is rather high compared to the standard error, basically the necessity of a random intercept has to be evaluated with the likelihood ratio test. The -2 log likelihood of a model with no random intercept appeared to be 1825.1 (results not shown in detail). The difference between the -2 log likelihoods is therefore 255.8, i.e. as expected highly significant. So, a random intercept is necessary in this particular situation.

The next step in the analysis is to add a random slope with time to the model. Output 7.6 shows the results of this random coefficient analysis. From Output 7.6, it can be seen that the log likelihood of a model with both a random intercept and a random slope with time is decreased (i.e. -774.78094).

Output 7.6. Result of a random coefficient analysis with a categorical outcome variable and both a random intercept and a random slope with time

```
log likelihood = -774.78094
------------------------------------------------------------------------------
      ycat      Coeff     Std. Err.      z     P > |z|    [95% Conf. Interval]
------------------------------------------------------------------------------
c2
        x1   -1.355226    1.601634    -0.846   0.397    -4.494371    1.783918
        x2    0.686692    0.1835857    3.740   0.000     0.3268706   1.046513
        x3    0.1369879   0.4222135    0.324   0.746    -0.6905353   0.9645111
        x4    0.4695151   0.8257442    0.569   0.570    -1.148914    2.087944
      time   -0.2982958   0.1261828   -2.364   0.018    -0.5456096  -0.050982
     _cons    1.529132    4.094066     0.373   0.709    -6.495091    9.553355
------------------------------------------------------------------------------
c3
        x1   -0.4861587   1.606773    -0.303   0.762    -3.635377    2.663059
        x2    1.013631    0.1828736    5.543   0.000     0.655205    1.372056
        x3   -0.1561199   0.4317889   -0.362   0.718    -1.002411    0.6901707
        x4    0.5955992   0.8259557    0.721   0.471    -1.023244    2.214443
      time   -0.3646409   0.1269982   -2.871   0.004    -0.6135529  -0.115729
     _cons   -1.372806    4.102624    -0.335   0.738    -9.413802    6.66819
------------------------------------------------------------------------------

Variances and covariances of random effects
------------------------------------------------------------------------------
***level 2 (id)
  var(1): 27.089896   (8.6944303)
cov(1,2): -2.9612643  (1.2660617)   cor(1,2): -0.85743581
  var(2): 0.44029501  (0.18979326)
```

With this value and the log likelihood value of a model with only a random intercept, the necessity of a random slope with time can be evaluated. The difference between the -2 log likelihoods of the both models is 19.72, which follows a χ^2 distribution with two degrees of freedom, i.e. highly significant. In other words, both a random intercept and a random slope with time must be considered.

7.2 'Count' outcome variables

A special type of categorical outcome variable is a so-called 'count' outcome variable (e.g. the number of asthma attacks in one year, the incidence rate of a specific disease, etc.). Because of the discrete and non-negative nature of the 'count' outcome variables, they are assumed to follow a Poisson distribution. Longitudinal analysis with 'count' outcome variables is therefore comparable to a (simple) Poisson regression analysis, the difference being that the longitudinal technique takes into account the within-subject correlations. It should further be noted that the longitudinal Poisson regression analysis is sometimes referred to as longitudinal log-linear regression analysis.

As for the longitudinal linear regression analysis, the longitudinal logistic regression analysis, and the longitudinal polytomous logistic regression analysis, the longitudinal Poisson regression analysis is, in fact, nothing more than an extension of the simple Poisson regression analysis; an extension which allows a within-subject correlation between the repeated measurements. With this analysis the development of the 'count' outcome variable can be related to several predictor variables, several time-dependent covariates, several time-independent covariates and time. As in (simple) cross-sectional Poisson regression analysis, all predictor variables and covariates can be continuous, dichotomous or categorical, although of course in the latter situation dummy coding can or must be used. As in (simple) cross-sectional Poisson regression analysis, the regression coefficient can be transformed into a rate ratio (exp(regression coefficient)). For estimation of the regression coefficients (i.e. rate ratios) the same sophisticated methods can be used as were discussed before, i.e. GEE analysis and random coefficient analysis. With GEE analysis, a correction for the within-subject correlations is made by assuming a 'working correlation structure', while with random coefficient analysis the different regression coefficients are allowed to vary between individuals (for technical details see for instance Diggle et al., 1994; Goldstein, 1995).

7.2.1 Example

7.2.1.1 Introduction

The example chosen to illustrate the analysis of a 'count' outcome variable is taken from the same longitudinal study which was used to illustrate most of the other techniques, i.e. the Amsterdam Growth and Health Longitudinal Study (Kemper, 1995). One of the aims of the presented study was to investigate the possible clustering of risk factors for coronary heart disease (CHD) and the longitudinal relationship with several 'lifestyle' predictor variables. To construct a measure of clustering, at each of the six measurements 'high risk' quartiles were formed for each of the following biological risk factors: (1) the ratio between total serum cholesterol and high density lipoprotein

Table 7.2. Number of subjects with a particular cluster score (i.e. the number of CHD risk factors) measured at six measurements

Time-point	Number of CHD risk factors				
	0	1	2	3	4
1	65	49	25	4	4
2	60	44	33	9	1
3	47	64	26	9	1
4	54	53	29	9	2
5	56	53	26	11	1
6	55	46	33	13	0

cholesterol, (2) diastolic blood pressure, (3) the sum of skinfolds, and (4) cardiopulmonary fitness. At each of the repeated measurements, clustering was defined as the number of biological risk factors that occurred in a particular subject. So, if a subject belonged to the 'high risk' quartile for all biological risk factors, the clustering score at that particular measurement was 4, if the subject belonged to three 'high risk' groups, the clustering score was 3, etc. This cluster score is a 'count' outcome variable, and this outcome variable Y_{count} is related to four predictor variables: (1) the baseline Keys score (a time-independent continuous variable), which is an indicator of the amount of unfavourable fatty acids and cholesterol in the diet, (2) the amount of physical activity (a time-dependent continuous variable), (3) smoking behaviour (a time-dependent dichotomous variable), and (4) gender (a time-independent dichotomous variable) (Twisk et al., 2001). In Tables 7.2 and 7.3 descriptive information about the example dataset is shown.

Again, the aim of this study was to investigate the longitudinal relationship between the four predictor variables and the clustering of CHD risk factors. In the example, both GEE analysis and random coefficient analysis will be used to investigate the longitudinal relationships.

7.2.1.2 GEE analysis

With 'count' outcome variables, the GEE approach also requires the choice of a working correlation structure. In principle, there are the same possibilities

Table 7.3. Descriptive information[a] about the predictor variables in the dataset with a 'count' outcome variable

Time-point	Keys score	Activity	Smoking	Gender
1	52.0 (7.9)	4.35 (1.9)	4/143	69/78
2	52.0 (7.9)	3.90 (1.6)	11/136	69/78
3	52.0 (7.9)	3.62 (1.7)	22/125	69/78
4	52.0 (7.9)	3.52 (1.8)	28/119	69/78
5	52.0 (7.9)	3.37 (2.1)	48/99	69/78
6	52.0 (7.9)	3.02 (2.1)	40/107	69/78

[a] For the Keys score and activity, mean and standard deviation are given; for smoking, the number of smokers/non-smokers is given; for gender, the number of males/females is given.

as have been discussed for continuous outcome variables (see Section 4.5.2). However, as for the dichotomous outcome variable, it can be problematic to use the correlation structure of the observed data as guidance for the choice of a working correlation structure. In this example, an exchangeable correlation structure will first be used.

Output 7.7 presents the results of the GEE analysis relating the longitudinal development of the outcome variable Y_{count} to the development of the four predictor variables. From the first line of Output 7.7 it can be seen that a 'Poisson' GEE analysis was performed, and from the second line of the

Output 7.7. Results of a GEE analysis with a 'count' outcome variable

```
Poisson Generalized Estimating Equations
Response: YCOUNT   Corr: Exchangeable
Column  Name      Coeff   StErr  p-value    IDR    95%     CI
----------------------------------------------------------------
   0    Constant   0.137  0.481   0.776
   2    TIME       0.004  0.021   0.856   1.004  0.963  1.046
   4    KEYS       0.002  0.008   0.806   1.002  0.987  1.017
   5    ACTIVITY  -0.084  0.021   0.000   0.920  0.882  0.959
   6    SMOKING    0.018  0.076   0.812   1.018  0.877  1.182
   7    GENDER     0.004  0.116   0.976   1.004  0.800  1.260
----------------------------------------------------------------
n:147   s:0.966   #iter:12
Estimate of common correlation 0.439
```

output it can be seen that an exchangeable correlation structure was used for estimation of the regression coefficients. As for all the other GEE outputs that have already been discussed, the next part of the output shows the parameter estimates, i.e. the regression coefficients, the standard errors of the regression coefficients and the p-values. Furthermore, the output gives the IDR and the corresponding 95% confidence intervals. The IDR is the 'incidence density ratio', which is equal to the rate ratio. The last two lines of the output give some additional information: the number of subjects ($n = 147$), the scale parameter ($s = 0.966$), the number of iterations needed to arrive at the given solution (#iter:12), and the estimate of the common (exchangeable) correlation coefficient (0.439).

As in the GEE analyses with a continuous and a dichotomous outcome variable, the scale parameter (also known as dispersion parameter) is an indication of the variance of the model. The interpretation of this coefficient is comparable to the interpretation of the scale parameter for a dichotomous outcome variable. This has to do with the characteristics of the Poisson distribution on which the Poisson GEE analysis is based. Within the Poisson distribution the variance is exactly the same as the mean value. So, for the Poisson GEE analysis, the scale parameter has to be one (i.e. a direct relationship between the variance and the mean). From Output 7.7, however, it can be seen that the scale parameter was slightly lower than one (i.e. 0.966). This phenomenon is sometimes referred to as underdispersion. When the scale parameter is greater than one, i.e. a situation which is much more common in practice, it is known as overdispersion. For a detailed technical description of this phenomenon, reference is made to for instance Lindsey (1993), Diggle et al. (1994), and Agresti et al. (2000). It should further be noted that in some software packages, the scale parameter for Poisson GEE analysis is set at a fixed value of one.

Looking at the estimated parameters, it can be seen that there is a highly significant inverse relationship between the CHD risk cluster score and the amount of physical activity, i.e. IDR = 0.92 with a 95% confidence interval from 0.88 to 0.96, and a highly significant p-value ($p < 0.001$). As for all other methods of longitudinal data analysis, this rate ratio can be interpreted in two ways: (1) a difference of one unit in physical activity between subjects is associated with a 9% ($1/0.92 = 1.09$) percent difference (i.e. lower) in the number of CHD risk factors (i.e the 'between-subjects' interpretation), and

Output 7.8. Results of GEE analyses with a 'count' outcome variable with an independent correlation structure (A), an 5-dependent correlation structure (B), and an unstructured correlation structure (C)

```
(A) Poisson Generalized Estimating Equations
Response: YCOUNT    Corr: Independence
Column   Name          Coeff    StErr    p-value      IDR      95%       CI
-----------------------------------------------------------------------------
   0     Constant      0.218    0.494    0.660
   2     TIME         -0.009    0.022    0.695      0.991    0.950     1.035
   4     KEYS          0.002    0.008    0.776      1.002    0.987     1.018
   5     ACTIVITY     -0.099    0.025    0.000      0.906    0.862     0.951
   6     SMOKING       0.138    0.103    0.181      1.148    0.938     1.404
   7     GENDER       -0.011    0.119    0.924      0.989    0.783     1.248
-----------------------------------------------------------------------------

n:147    s:0.966    #iter:11

(B) Poisson Generalized Estimating Equations
Response: YCOUNT    Corr: 5-Dependence
Column   Name          Coeff    StErr    p-value      IDR      95%       CI
-----------------------------------------------------------------------------
   0     Constant      0.123    0.487    0.801
   2     TIME          0.004    0.021    0.859      1.004    0.964     1.045
   4     KEYS          0.002    0.008    0.792      1.002    0.987     1.018
   5     ACTIVITY     -0.083    0.019    0.000      0.921    0.887     0.956
   6     SMOKING       0.040    0.072    0.584      1.040    0.903     1.198
   7     GENDER       -0.001    0.117    0.996      0.999    0.795     1.257
-----------------------------------------------------------------------------

n:147    s:0.967    #iter:12
Estimate of common correlations 0.543, 0.451, 0.427, 0.383, 0.279

(C) Poisson Generalized Estimating Equations
Response: YCOUNT    Corr: Unspecified
Column   Name          Coeff    StErr    p-value      IDR      95%       CI
-----------------------------------------------------------------------------
   0     Constant      0.132    0.481    0.783
   2     TIME          0.009    0.020    0.660      1.009    0.970     1.049
   4     KEYS          0.002    0.008    0.843      1.002    0.987     1.017
   5     ACTIVITY     -0.077    0.019    0.000      0.926    0.893     0.960
   6     SMOKING       0.018    0.072    0.806      1.018    0.883     1.173
   7     GENDER       -0.010    0.116    0.929      0.990    0.789     1.242
-----------------------------------------------------------------------------

n:147    s:0.968    #iter:12

Estimate of common correlation
1.000    0.587    0.536    0.483    0.362    0.257
0.587    1.000    0.537    0.554    0.455    0.352
0.536    0.537    1.000    0.562    0.418    0.300
0.483    0.554    0.562    1.000    0.429    0.280
0.362    0.455    0.418    0.429    1.000    0.550
0.257    0.352    0.300    0.280    0.550    1.000
```

Table 7.4. Results of GEE analyses with a 'count' outcome variable with different correlation structures

	Correlation structure			
	Independent	Exchangeable	5-Dependent	Unstructured
Keys score	0.00 (0.01)	0.00 (0.01)	0.00 (0.01)	0.00 (0.01)
Activity	−0.10 (0.03)	−0.08 (0.02)	−0.08 (0.02)	−0.08 (0.02)
Smoking	0.14 (0.10)	0.02 (0.08)	0.04 (0.07)	0.02 (0.07)
Gender	−0.01 (0.12)	0.00 (0.12)	0.00 (0.12)	−0.01 (0.12)
Time	−0.01 (0.02)	0.00 (0.02)	0.00 (0.02)	0.01 (0.02)

(2) a change of one unit in physical activity within a subject (over a certain time period) is associated with a decrease of 9% in the number of CHD risk factors (i.e the 'within-subject' interpretation).

As has been mentioned for the linear and the logistic GEE analysis, an alternative model (i.e. an autoregressive model) can be used to obtain an estimate for the 'within-subject' relationship. The procedures are the same as those described in Chapter 5, so this will not be further discussed.

To investigate the influence of using a different correlation structure, the data were re-analysed with an independent, a 5-dependent, and an unstructured correlation structure. The results are presented in Output 7.8, and in Table 7.4 the results of the Poisson GEE analyses with different correlation structures are summarized.

From Table 7.4 it can be seen that the differences between the results are only marginal. In fact, the results obtained from the GEE analysis with the three dependent (i.e. exchangeable, 5-depenendent and unstructured) correlation structures are almost the same. This was also observed for the GEE analysis with a dichotomous outcome variable. In other words, for the longitudinal analysis of a 'count' outcome variable, GEE analysis also seems to be quite robust against a 'wrong' choice of a 'working correlation structure'. For the analysis with an independent correlation structure, the regression coefficients are slightly different than for the analysis with the three dependent correlation structures, and the standard errors are slightly higher for all predictor variables. For the time-dependent predictor variables this difference was, however, more pronounced than for the time-independent predictor variables. This is exactly the same as has been observed for dichotomous outcome variables (see Section 6.2.4.1), but differs from the GEE analysis with continuous outcome variables (see Section 4.5.4.3).

7.2.1.3 Random coefficient analysis

The first random coefficient analysis performed on this dataset is an analysis with only a random intercept. Output 7.9 shows the result of this random coefficient analysis. The output of the random coefficient analysis looks the same as the output that has been discussed earlier for continuous outcome

Output 7.9. Results of a random coefficient analysis with a 'count' outcome variable and only a random intercept

```
Random-effects Poisson                  Number of obs       =        882
Group variable (i) : id                 Number of groups    =        147
Random effects u_i ~ Gaussian           Obs per group: min  =          6
                                                       avg  =        6.0
                                                       max  =          6
                                        LR chi2(5)          =      15.80
Log likelihood = -1051.444              Prob > chi2         =     0.0074
-----------------------------------------------------------------------------
   YCOUNT      Coeff    Std. Err.      z     P>|z|    [95% Conf. Interval]
-----------------------------------------------------------------------------
     KEYS   0.0037919  0.0081538    0.465   0.642   -0.0121892    0.0197731
 ACTIVITY  -0.0885626  0.0242515   -3.652   0.000   -0.1360946   -0.0410306
  SMOKING   0.0398486  0.1112441    0.358   0.720   -0.1781858    0.257883
   GENDER  -0.0312362  0.1298678   -0.241   0.810   -0.2857725    0.2233
     TIME   0.0021113  0.0218432    0.097   0.923   -0.0407005    0.0449231
    _cons  -0.0706359  0.5193567   -0.136   0.892   -1.088556     0.9472846
-----------------------------------------------------------------------------
 /lnsig2u  -0.9209769  0.215503    -4.274   0.000   -1.343355    -0.4985988
-----------------------------------------------------------------------------
  sigma_u   0.6309754  0.0679886                     0.5108509    0.7793466
      rho   0.2847589  0.0438918                     0.2069589    0.37787
-----------------------------------------------------------------------------
Likelihood ratio test of rho=0:  chi2(1) = 124.50   Prob > chi2 = 0.0000
```

variables and dichotomous outcome variables. The first part contains general information about the model. It shows that a Poisson random coefficient analysis was performed (Random-effects Poisson) and that the random coefficients are normally distributed (Random effects u_i ~ Gaussian). It also shows the log likelihood of the model and the result of a likelihood ratio test (LR chi2(5) = 15.80). This likelihood ratio test is related to the comparison between this model and a model with a random intercept but without predictor variables. Because five predictor variables are analysed (time, Keys score, activity, smoking and gender), the difference between the two -2 log likelihoods follows a χ^2 distribution with five degrees of freedom. The corresponding p-value is prob > chi2 = 0.0074, which is highly significant.

The second part of the output shows information about the (fixed) regression coefficients. First of all, the regression coefficients can be transformed into rate ratios by taking exp(coef), and secondly the interpretation of the regression coefficients is the same as has been discussed for the GEE analysis with the 'count' outcome variable. So again, the interpretation is a combination of a 'between-subjects' (cross-sectional) interpretation and a 'within-subject' (longitudinal) interpretation.

The last part of the output shows information about the random part of the analysis. It includes the variance of the (normally distributed) random intercepts (sigma_u) and the estimate of the within-subject correlation (rho). Furthermore, the natural log of sigma_u is shown (/lnsig2u), although this information is not really interesting.

The result of the likelihood ratio test of rho = 0 is based on the comparison between the presented model and a model with no random intercept, but with all predictor variables included. This difference is 124.50, and it follows a χ^2 distribution with one degree of freedom (i.e. the random intercept). The corresponding p-value (prob > chi2) is very low (i.e. highly significant), so it is necessary to allow a random intercept.

The next step in the analysis is to investigate the necessity of allowing a random slope with time as well. Therefore, a random coefficient analysis with both a random intercept and a random slope with time is performed. The result of this analysis is shown in Output 7.10.

To investigate the need for a random slope with time (in addition to the random intercept), the log likelihood of the model with only a random intercept can be compared to the log likelihood of the model with both a random intercept and a random slope with time. The difference between these log likelihoods is 1.2638. Because the likelihood ratio test is based on the difference between the -2 log likelihoods, the calculated difference has

Output 7.10. Result of a random coefficient analysis with a 'count' outcome variable and both a random intercept and a random slope with time

```
log likelihood = -1050.1802
-------------------------------------------------------------------------------
  YCOUNT     Coeff     Std. Err.      z      P > |z|     [95% Conf. Interval]
-------------------------------------------------------------------------------
    KEYS    0.0037276  0.0080096   0.465    0.642    -0.0119709    0.0194261
ACTIVITY   -0.0862816  0.0242208  -3.562    0.000    -0.1337535   -0.0388097
 SMOKING    0.0338785  0.1082511   0.313    0.754    -0.1782898    0.2460467
  GENDER   -0.0184725  0.1281452  -0.144    0.885    -0.2696325    0.2326876
    TIME    0.0275027  0.0273572   1.005    0.315    -0.0261163    0.0811218
   _cons   -0.1889464  0.5126143  -0.369    0.712    -1.193652     0.8157592
-------------------------------------------------------------------------------

Variances and covariances of random effects
-------------------------------------------------------------------------------
***level 2 (id)
  var(1):   0.61590233 (0.19406681)
cov(1,2): -0.03402709 (0.02612385) cor(1,2): -1
  var(2):   0.00187991 (0.00236976)
```

to be multiplied by two. This value (i.e. 2.5276) follows a χ^2 distribution with two degrees of freedom (i.e the random slope with time and the covariance between the random intercept and random slope). The corresponding p-value is 0.28, which is not significant, so a random slope with time is not necessary in this situation.

7.2.2 Comparison between GEE analysis and random coefficient analysis

In Table 7.5, the results of the longitudinal analysis with a 'count' outcome variable performed with GEE analysis and random coefficient analysis are summarized. When the results of the GEE analysis and the random coefficient analysis are compared, it can be concluded that the differences observed for dichotomous outcome variables are not observed for a 'count' outcome variable. In fact, the observed differences between the two sophisticated techniques are only marginal, although both the regression coefficients and the standard errors obtained from the random coefficient analysis are, in general, slightly higher than those obtained from the GEE analysis. The fact that the 'subject-specific' regression coefficients and standard errors are slightly

Table 7.5. Regression coefficients and standard errors (in parentheses) of longitudinal regression analyses with a 'count' outcome variable; a comparison between GEE analysis and random coefficient analysis

	GEE analysis[a]	Random coefficient analysis[b]
Keys score	0.00 (0.01)	0.00 (0.01)
Activity	−0.08 (0.02)	−0.09 (0.02)
Smoking	0.02 (0.08)	0.04 (0.11)
Gender	0.00 (0.12)	−0.03 (0.13)
Time	0.00 (0.02)	0.00 (0.02)

[a] GEE analysis with an exchangeable correlation structure.
[b] Random coefficient analysis with only a random intercept.

higher than the 'population-averaged' regression coefficients has to do with the characteristics of the log-linear model compared to the linear model. However, the differences are far less pronounced than has been discussed for the logistic model.

Longitudinal studies with two measurements: the definition and analysis of change

8.1 Introduction

In the foregoing chapters various sophisticated methods to analyse the longitudinal relationships between an outcome variable Y and several predictor variables X have been discussed. In the examples, a dataset with six measurements was used to illustrate the specific techniques and to demonstrate the use of particular models for longitudinal data analyses. All the methods that have been discussed are also suitable for use in studies in which only two measurements are carried out. However, with only two measurements the more sophisticated statistical techniques are (unfortunately) seldom or never applied. In practice, in studies with only two measurements, the longitudinal problem is often reduced to a cross-sectional one, i.e. a problem for which (simple) cross-sectional statistical techniques can be used. One of the methods that is most frequently used to analyse longitudinal relationships in studies with two measurements is the analysis of change. The change in outcome variable Y is related to the change in one or more predictor variables X. In this chapter, several ways in which to define changes between subsequent measurements will be discussed. The way change can or must be defined is highly dependent on the structure of the variable of interest, and on the research questions to be addressed. Like in most other chapters, separate sections will deal with continuous outcome variables and dichotomous and categorical outcome variables.

8.2 Continuous outcome variables

The relationship between a change in a continuous outcome variable and (changes in) several predictor variables can be analysed by simple linear regression analysis. This is a very popular method, which greatly reduces the complexity of the statistical analysis. However, how to define the change between two repeated measurements is often more complicated than is usually realized.

In the literature, several methods with which to define changes in continuous outcome variables have been reported. The simplest method is to calculate the absolute difference between two measurements over time (Equation (8.1)), a method that is also used in the paired t-test and in the MANOVA for repeated measurements (see Chapter 3).

$$\Delta Y = Y_{it2} - Y_{it1} \tag{8.1}$$

where Y_{it2} are observations for subject i at time t_2, and Y_{it1} are observations for subject i at time t_1.

In some situations it is possible that the relative difference between two subsequent measurements is a better estimate of the 'real' change (Equation (8.2)):

$$\Delta Y = \frac{(Y_{it2} - Y_{it1})}{Y_{it1}} \times 100\% \tag{8.2}$$

where Y_{it2} are observations for subject i at time t_2 and Y_{it1} are observations for subject i at time t_1.

Both techniques are suitable in situations in which the continuous outcome variable theoretically ranges from 0 to $+\infty$, or from $-\infty$ to 0, or from $-\infty$ to $+\infty$. Some variables (e.g. scores on questionnaires) have maximal possible values ('ceilings') and/or minimal possible values ('floors'). To take these 'ceilings' and/or 'floors' into account, the definition of change can be as shown in Equation (8.3).

$$\text{when } Y_{it2} > Y_{it1}: \quad \Delta Y = \frac{(Y_{it2} - Y_{it1})}{(Y_{\max} - Y_{it1})} \times 100\% \tag{8.3a}$$

$$\text{when } Y_{it2} < Y_{it1}: \quad \Delta Y = \frac{(Y_{it2} - Y_{it1})}{(Y_{it1} - Y_{\min})} \times 100\% \tag{8.3b}$$

$$\text{when } Y_{it2} = Y_{it1}: \quad \Delta Y = 0 \tag{8.3c}$$

where Y_{it2} are observations for subject i at time t_2, Y_{it1} are observations for subject i at time t_1, $Y_{\max}$ is the maximal possible value of Y ('ceiling'), and $Y_{\min}$ is the minimal possible value of Y ('floor').

It is sometimes suggested to apply Equation (8.4) to take into account possible 'floor' or 'ceiling' effects.

$$\Delta Y = \frac{(Y_{it2} - Y_{it1})}{(Y_{max} - Y_{min})} \times 100\% \tag{8.4}$$

where Y_{it2} are observations for subject i at time t_2, Y_{it1} are observations for subject i at time t_1, Y_{max} is the maximal possible value of Y ('ceiling'), and Y_{min} is the minimal possible value of Y ('floor'). However, Equation (8.4) is nothing more than a linear transformation of the absolute difference (i.e. divided by the range and multiplied by 100). So, basically, the definition of change based on Equation (8.4) does not take into account possible 'floors' or 'ceilings'.

One of the typical problems related to the definitions of change discussed so far is the phenomenon of regression to the mean. If the outcome variable at $t = 1$ is a sample of random numbers, and the outcome variable at $t = 2$ is also a sample of random numbers, then the subjects in the upper part of the distribution at $t = 1$ are less likely to be in the upper part of the distribution at $t = 2$, compared to the other subjects. In the same way, the subjects in the lower part of the distribution at $t = 1$ are less likely than the other subjects to be in the lower part of the distribution at $t = 2$. The consequence of this is that, just by chance, the change between $t = 1$ and $t = 2$ is (highly) related to the initial value.

There are, however, some ways in which it is possible to define changes between subsequent measurements, more or less 'correcting' for the phenomenon of regression to the mean. One of these approaches is known as 'analysis of covariance' (Equation (8.5)). With this technique the value of the outcome variable Y at the second measurement is used as outcome variable in a linear regression analysis, with the observation of the outcome variable Y at the first measurement as one of the predictor variables (i.e. as a covariate):

$$Y_{it2} = \beta_0 + \beta_1 Y_{it1} + \cdots + \varepsilon_i \tag{8.5}$$

where Y_{it2} are observations for subject i at time t_2, Y_{it1} are observations for subject i at time t_1, and ε_i is the 'error' for subject i.

Other predictor variables can be added to this linear regression model. This analysis of covariance is almost, but not quite, the same as the calculation of the 'absolute' difference (see Equation (8.1)). This can be seen when Equation (8.5) is written as Equation (8.6).

$$Y_{it2} - \beta_1 Y_{it1} = \beta_0 + \cdots + \varepsilon_i \qquad (8.6)$$

where Y_{it2} are observations for subject i at time t_2, Y_{it1} are observations for subject i at time t_1, and ε_i is the 'error' of subject i.

In the analysis of covariance, the change is defined **relative** to the value of Y at $t = 1$. This relativity is expressed in the regression coefficient β_1, which is known as the autoregression coefficient (see also Section 5.2.3), and therefore it is assumed that this method 'corrects' for the phenomenon of regression to the mean. This analysis is comparable to the analysis of 'residual change', which was first described by Blomquist (1977). The first step in this method is to perform a linear regression analysis between Y_{t2} and Y_{t1} (Equation (8.5)). The second step is to calculate the difference between the observed value of Y_{t2} and the predicted value of Y_{t2} (predicted by the regression model described in Equation (8.5)). This difference is called the 'residual change', which is then used as outcome variable in a linear regression analysis in which the relationship between the changes in several variables can be analysed.

Some researchers argue that the best way to define changes, correcting for the phenomenon of regression to the mean, is a combination of Equations (8.1) and (8.5). They suggest calculating the absolute change between Y_{t2} and Y_{t1}, correcting for the value of Y_{t1} (Equation (8.7)).

$$Y_{it2} - Y_{it1} = \beta_0 + \beta_1 Y_{it1} + \cdots + \varepsilon_i \qquad (8.7)$$

where Y_{it2} are observations for subject i at time t_2, Y_{it1} are observations for subject i at time t_1, and ε_i is the 'error' of subject i.

However, analysing the change, correcting for the initial value at $t = 1$, is exactly the same as the analysis of covariance described in Equation (8.5). This can be seen when Equation (8.7) is written in another way (Equation (8.8)). The only difference between the models is that the regression coefficient for the initial value is different, i.e. the difference between the regression coefficients for the initial value is equal to one.

$$Y_{it2} = \beta_0 + (\beta_1 + 1) \, Y_{it1} + \cdots + \varepsilon_i \qquad (8.8)$$

Table 8.1. Part of the example dataset used to illustrate the phenomenon of regression to the mean

ID	Y_{t1}	Y_{t2}	$Y_{t2} - Y_{t1}$	Pred $(Y_{t2})^a$	Residual change[b]
1	4.2	3.9	−0.30	4.14786	0.25
2	4.4	4.2	−0.20	4.29722	0.10
3	3.7	4.0	0.30	3.77447	−0.23
⋮					
147	4.6	4.4	−0.20	4.44658	0.05

[a] Predicted by the regression equation $Y_{t2} = \beta_0 + \beta_1 Y_{t1}$.
[b] Calculated as Y_{t2} minus the predicted value of Y_{t2}.

where Y_{it2} are observations for subject i at time t_2, Y_{it1} are observations for subject i at time t_1, and ε_i is the 'error' of subject i.

Because it is sometimes difficult to understand what the assumed correction for the phenomenon of regression to the mean really implies, the following section presents a numerical example to illustrate this phenomenon.

8.2.1 A numerical example

The illustration is based on the first two measurements of the example dataset. Table 8.1 shows part of the dataset. To illustrate the phenomenon of regression to the mean, the population is divided into two groups. The groups are based on the median of Y_{t1}; the upper half is coded as '1', the lower half is coded as '0'. This dichotomous group indicator is now related to the change in outcome variable Y between $t = 2$ and $t = 1$. This change is defined in four ways: (1) absolute change (Equation (8.1)), (2) residual change, (3) analysis of covariance (Equation (8.5)), and (4) absolute change, correcting for the initial value of Y (Equation (8.7)). In Output 8.1, the results of the different regression analyses are presented.

The results shown in Output 8.1 are quite clear. The absolute change in outcome variable Y between $t = 2$ and $t = 1$ is highly associated with the group indicator. The change in the outcome variable Y between $t = 1$ and $t = 2$ in the upper half of the distribution at $t = 1$ is 0.287 higher than the change in the lower half of the distribution. When the analysis of residual change or the analysis of covariance is applied, however, the effect of

Output 8.1. Results of several linear regression analyses relating the change in outcome variable Y between $t = 1$ and $t = 2$ to a group indicator based on the median of Y_{t1}; (A) absolute change, (B) residual change, (C) analysis of covariance, (D) absolute change, correcting for the initial value of Y

(A)	B	Std. error	Standardized coefficient	t	Sig
Constant	0.002	0.051		0.456	0.649
Group	-0.287	0.074	-0.307	-3.881	0.000

Dependent variable: Difference between initial value and follow-up

(B)	B	Std. error	Standardized coefficient	t	Sig
Constant	0.000	0.050		-0.175	0.861
Group	0.002	0.072	0.021	0.255	0.799

Dependent variable: Residual change

(C)	B	Std. error	Standardized coefficient	t	Sig
Constant	0.908	0.348		2.608	0.010
Group	-0.005	0.118	-0.037	-0.413	0.680
Initial value	0.775	0.088	0.785	8.859	0.000

Dependent variable: Follow-up value

(D)	B	Std. error	Standardized coefficient	t	Sig
Constant	0.908	0.348		2.608	0.010
Group	-0.005	0.118	-0.037	-0.413	0.680
Initial value	-0.225	0.088	-0.323	-2.568	0.011

Dependent variable: Difference between baseline and follow-up

belonging to the upper or lower half of the distribution totally disappears. It is also shown that the analysis of absolute change, correcting for the initial value, is exactly the same as the analysis of covariance. The only difference is observed in the regression coefficient for the baseline value: a difference that is equal to one (see also Equation (8.8)).

Table 8.2. Mean and standard deviation (in parentheses) for the variables used in the present example

	t_1	t_2 (after 26 weeks)
Barthel index	6.6 (4.0)	16.0 (4.8)
Age (in years)	64.1 (12.9)	
Gender (males/females)	24/21	

Although this example seems to be extreme, such situations do occur. Suppose that a population-based intervention is applied (e.g. a population-based dietary intervention), in order to decrease cholesterol concentrations in the blood. Suppose further that the hypothesis is that the intervention is highly successful for the subjects with the highest cholesterol levels at baseline. Owing to the phenomenon of regression to the mean, the intervention will (indeed) be highly successful for the subjects with the highest cholesterol levels at baseline. However, the question remains whether this is a real effect or an artefact.

8.2.2 Example

The dataset used to illustrate the different possible ways in which to define change differs from that used for the other examples. This dataset has an outcome variable in which 'floor' and 'ceiling' effects can be illustrated. It is derived from a study performed by Kwakkel et al. (1999), in which the change in physical function after stroke was investigated. Physical function was measured according to the Barthel index, which measures a patient's ability to carry out ten everyday tasks. This index (the outcome variable) is assumed continuous, and can range between 0 and 20. The outcome variable is measured in the same subjects ($N = 45$) on two occasions over time (with a time interval of 26 weeks). Changes between the subsequent measurements are related to two predictor variables measured at baseline: age (a continuous predictor variable) and gender (a dichotomous predictor variable). Table 8.2 gives descriptive information about the variables used in the present example.

To define the change in outcome variable Y between t_1 and t_2, three methods were used based on (1) the absolute difference (Equation (8.1)),

Table 8.3. Mean and standard deviation for the 'change' variables used in the example

	Mean	Standard deviation
(1) Absolute change	9.4	3.7
(2) Relative change (%)[a]	247.2	244.4
(3) Change taking into account 'ceiling' (%)	75.3	28.4

[a] Because the relative change value was highly skewed to the right, a natural log transformation was carried out before the regression analysis was performed.

Table 8.4. Regression coefficients and standard errors (in parentheses) of linear regression analyses with different approaches to defining change

	Age	Gender
(1) Absolute change	−0.065 (0.043)	−0.17 (1.11)
(2) Relative change	0.005 (0.012)	−0.09 (0.31)
(3) Change taking into account 'ceiling'	−0.862 (0.310)	7.69 (7.96)
(4) Analysis of residual change	−0.079 (0.042)	0.06 (1.07)
(5) Analysis of covariance	−0.085 (0.043)	0.15 (1.09)
(6) Absolute change (correcting for Y at t_1)	−0.085 (0.043)	0.15 (1.09)

(2) the relative difference (Equation (8.2)), and (3) the difference taking into account the 'ceiling' of the outcome variable Y (Equation (8.3)). Table 8.3 gives descriptive information about the three 'change' variables.

All three differences were related to the two predictor variables with simple linear (cross-sectional) regression analysis. Also applied were the analysis of residual change, the analysis of covariance (Equation (8.5)), and the approach in which the absolute change is related to the two predictor variables, correcting for the value of Y at t_1 (Equation (8.7)). Table 8.4 presents the results of the different regression analyses.

The purpose of this example is not to decide what is the best way in which to define change in this particular example; this choice should be (mainly) based on biological considerations. The important message from the example is that the definition of change greatly influences the results of the analyses, and therefore greatly influences the answer to the research question.

8.3 Dichotomous and categorical outcome variables

For dichotomous outcome variables the situation is slightly more difficult than was described for continuous outcome variables. This is due to the fact that a change in a dichotomous outcome variable between subsequent measurements leads to a categorical variable. First of all, there are subjects who stay in the 'highest' category, there are subjects who stay in the 'lowest' category, and there are subjects who move from one category to another (see Figure 6.2).

In general, for categorical outcome variables with C categories, the change between subsequent measurements is another categorical variable with C^2 categories. The cross-sectional analysis of the resulting categorical variable can be performed with polytomous/multinomial logistic regression analysis, which is now available in most software packages.

Unfortunately, polytomous logistic regression analysis is not much used. Therefore, in many studies the resulting categorical outcome variable is reduced to a dichotomous outcome variable, which can be analysed with simple logistic regression analysis. One widely used possibility is to discriminate between subjects who showed an 'increase' and subjects who did not, etc. Nevertheless, in every reduction information is lost, and it is obvious that a dichotomization is not recommended in most research situations.

Another method with which to analyse changes in a dichotomous outcome variable is analysis of covariance (see Equation (8.5)). Instead of a linear regression analysis, logistic regression analysis must be used for the dichotomous outcome variable.

8.3.1 Example

The example to illustrate the definition of change in a dichotomous outcome variable is based on the same dataset that has been used in the example with a continuous outcome variable. The research question to be addressed is also the same as has been answered for a continuous outcome variable: 'What is the relationship beteen age at baseline and gender and the changes in Barthel index over a period of 26 weeks?'

To create a dichotomous outcome variable, an arbitrary cut-off value for the Barthel index was chosen, i.e. subjects with a Barthel index >10 and

Table 8.5. Number of subjects with a Barthel index >10 and number of subjects with a Barthel index ≤ 10 at each of the repeated measurements

	t_1	t_2 (after 26 weeks)
Barthel index >10	9	37
Barthel index ≤ 10	36	8

Table 8.6. Regression coefficients[a] and standard errors (in parentheses) of polytomous logistic regression analysis and (logistic) analysis of covariance

	Age	Gender
(1) Polytomous logistic regression[b]		
Subjects staying in the highest category	−0.10 (0.05)	1.48 (1.16)
Subjects moving from the lowest to the		
highest category	−0.05 (0.05)	0.31 (0.85)
(2) (Logistic) analysis of covariance	−0.05 (0.05)	0.36 (0.85)

[a] The regression coefficients can be transformed to odds ratios by taking exp(regression coefficient).

[b] Staying in the lowest category is used as reference category.

subjects with a Barthel index ≤ 10. Table 8.5 gives descriptive information about this dichotomous outcome variable at each of the repeated measurements.

Because all subjects in the example dataset show an increase in their daily functioning (i.e. there is an increase in their Barthel index), the changes in the dichotomous outcome variable result in three groups: (1) subjects who stay in the lowest category ($N = 8$), (2) subjects who move from the lowest category to the highest category ($N = 28$), and (3) subjects who stay in the highest category ($N = 9$). This categorical 'change' variable can be analysed with polytomous (nominal) logistic regression. In addition a logistic analysis of covariance is also used to answer the research question. The results of both analyses are summarized in Table 8.6.

It is important to realize that the results of the (logistic) analysis of covariance are (almost) equal to the results of the comparison between subjects who stayed in the lowest category and subjects who moved from the lowest category to the highest category, obtained from the polytomous logistic regression analysis. So, both analyses basically provide the same information, although the polytomous logistic regression analysis is more extensive, because it provides additional information from a comparison between subjects who stayed in the highest category and subjects who stayed in the lowest category. However, it should be noted that this is only true in the present example in which there were no subjects moving from the highest to the lowest category. When the latter situation is also present, the interpretation of the logistic analysis of covariance can be very complicated and can easily lead to wrong conclusions.

8.4 Comments

In Chapter 5, several alternative methods to model longitudinal relationships were discussed. One of those methods dealt with the changes between subsequent measurements as units of analyses (see Section 5.2.2). For the definition of those changes the same problems arise as in the more simple situation in which there are only two measurements over time. Another problem with the modelling of changes between two consecutive measurements is the fact that the deviation in the result variable can be so small that it is difficult to detect any significant relationships. This is especially problematic when the time periods between the repeated measurements are short, or when the absolute value of the variable of interest is stable over time, i.e. when there is almost no change in the variable of interest over time.

Although the absolute change between two repeated measurements is often used to define changes between subsequent measurements, this method is often criticized; first of all because of its assumed negative correlation with the initial value (i.e. the phenomenon of regression to the mean), and secondly because of its low reliability. For more information on this issue, reference is made to Rogossa (1995) who gives an interesting overview of the 'myths and methods' in longitudinal research and, in particular, the definition of change. Furthermore, one must realize that statistical techniques like the paired t-test and MANOVA for repeated measurements (see Chapter 3) are methods that are based on the absolute change, and therefore have the same limitations as have been discussed in this chapter.

8.5 Sophisticated analyses

In a situation with two measurements, the sophisticated longitudinal techniques discussed in earlier chapters (i.e. GEE analysis and random coefficient analysis) can also be used. However, the results of these sophisticated analyses differ in an essential way from the results based on different definitions of change presented earlier. This is because the regression coefficients derived from GEE analysis and random coefficient analysis combine the information of the 'between-subjects' (cross-sectional) and 'within-subject' (longitudinal) relationships (see Section 4.5.2). In contrast, the (simple) analyses of change presented in this chapter investigate only the 'longitudinal' aspect of the relationship.

8.6 Conclusions

It is difficult to give straightforward advice regarding the definition of change that should be used in a longitudinal study with two measurements. The choice for a particular method greatly depends on the research questions to be addressed and the characteristics of the outcome variable. However, when a continuous outcome variable is involved and there are no anticipated 'ceiling' or 'floor' effects, the analysis of residual change or analysis of covariance is recommended, because both techniques correct (if necessary) for the phenomenon of regression to the mean. Although these two techniques both produce almost the same results, the analysis of covariance is probably the preferred method, because the regression coefficients of the final regression analysis are somewhat easier to interpret. When there are anticipated 'ceiling' or 'floor' effects, they should be taken into account. However, the best way of analysing change is (probably) a combination of the results of several analyses obtained from various (biologically plausible) definitions of change.

When changes in a dichotomous outcome variable are analysed, polytomous logistic regression analysis of the categorical variable is preferable to (logistic) analysis of covariance, because it provides more information and the interpretation of the results is fairly straightforward.

Analysis of experimental studies

9.1 Introduction

Experimental (longitudinal) studies differ from observational longitudinal studies in that experimental studies (in epidemiology often described as trials) include one or more interventions. In general, at baseline the population is (randomly) divided into two or more groups. In the case of two groups, one of the groups receives the intervention of interest and the other group receives a placebo intervention, no intervention at all, or the 'usual' treatment. Both groups are monitored over a certain period of time, in order to find out whether the groups differ with regard to a particular outcome variable. The outcome variable can be continuous, dichotomous or categorical.

In epidemiology, the simplest form of experimental longitudinal study is one in which a baseline measurement and only one follow-up measurement are performed (Figure 9.1). If the subjects are randomly assigned to the different groups (interventions), a comparison of the follow-up values between the groups will give an answer to the question of which intervention is more effective with regard to the particular outcome variable. The assumption is that random allocation at baseline will ensure that there is no difference between the groups at baseline (in fact, in this situation a baseline measure is not even necessary).

Another possibility is to analyse the changes between the values of the baseline and the follow-up measurement, and to compare these changes among the different groups. In Chapter 8 it was explained that the definition of change can be rather complicated and, although this technique is widely used to analyse experimental studies, the interpretation of the results is more difficult than many researchers think.

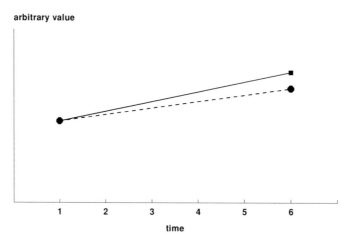

Figure 9.1. An experimental longitudinal study in which one intervention and one placebo
group are compared with regard to a continuous outcome variable at one
follow-up measurement (■ —— intervention, • – – – placebo).

In the past decade, experimental studies with only one follow-up measurement have become very rare. At least one short-term follow-up measurement
and one long-term follow-up measurement 'must' be performed. However,
more than two follow-up measurements are usually performed in order to
investigate the 'development' of the outcome variable, and to compare the
'developments' among the groups (Figure 9.2). These more complicated
experimental designs are often analysed with the simple methods that have
already been described, mostly by analysing the outcome at each follow-up
measurement separately, or sometimes even by ignoring the information
gathered from the in-between measurements, i.e. only using the last measurement as outcome variable to evaluate the effect of the intervention. This
is even more surprising, in view of the fact that there are statistical methods
available which can be used to analyse the difference in 'development' of the
outcome variable in two or more groups.

It is obvious that the methods that can be used for the statistical analysis
of experimental (longitudinal) studies are exactly the same as have been discussed for observational longitudinal studies. The remainder of this chapter
is devoted to an extensive example covering all aspects of the analysis of an
experimental study. For educational purposes, 'all' various possible ways to

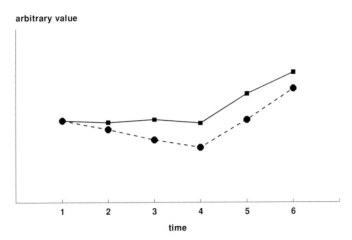

Figure 9.2. An experimental longitudinal study in which one intervention and one placebo group are compared with regard to a continuous outcome variable at more than one follow-up measurement (■ —— intervention, • – – – placebo).

analyse the data of an experimental study will be discussed. It should be realized that this will also include methods that are not really suitable in the situation of the example datasets.

9.2 Example with a continuous outcome variable

9.2.1 Introduction

The dataset used to illustrate an experimental study is (of course) different to the dataset used in the examples for observational longitudinal studies. The present example makes use of a dataset in which a therapy intervention is compared to a placebo intervention with regard to the development of systolic blood pressure (Vermeulen et al., 2000). In this experimental study, three measurements were carried out: one baseline measurement and two follow-up measurements with equally spaced time intervals. A total of 152 patients were included in the study, equally divided between the therapy and the placebo group.

Table 9.1 gives descriptive information about the variables used in the study, while Figure 9.3 illustrates the development of systolic blood pressure over time. The main aim of the therapy under study was not to lower the

Table 9.1. Mean and standard deviation (in parentheses) in the treatment groups at three time-points

	Placebo group			Therapy group		
	t_1	t_2	t_3	t_1	t_2	t_3
N	71	74	66	68	69	65
Systolic blood pressure	130.7	129.1	126.3	126.5	122.5	121.6
	(17.6)	(16.9)	(14.2)	(12.5)	(11.2)	(12.1)

systolic blood pressure

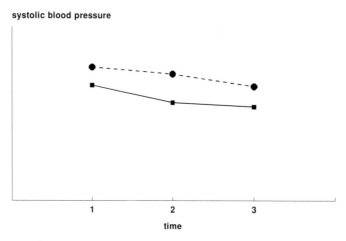

Figure 9.3. Development of systolic blood pressure over time in the treatment groups (■ —— therapy, • – – – placebo).

systolic blood pressure; this was investigated as a side-effect. That is one of the reasons why the number of subjects at baseline was lower than the number of subjects at the first follow-up measurement.

9.2.2 Simple analysis

The simplest way to answer the question of whether the therapy intervention is more effective than the placebo intervention is to compare systolic blood pressure values at the two follow-up measurements between the two groups. The hypothesis is that the systolic blood pressure will be lower in the group that received the therapy intervention than in the group that received the

Table 9.2. Mean systolic blood pressure at $t = 2$ and $t = 3$; a comparison between therapy and placebo group and p-values derived from independent sample t-tests

	Therapy	Placebo	p-Value
Short-term (systolic blood pressure at $t = 2$)	122.5	129.1	0.007
Long-term (systolic blood pressure at $t = 3$)	121.6	126.3	0.044

placebo intervention. In this example, a distinction can be made between the short-term effects and the long-term effects. To analyse the short-term effects, the mean systolic blood pressure measured at $t = 2$ can be compared between the therapy group and placebo group. For the long-term effects, the systolic blood pressure measured at $t = 3$ can be compared. The differences between the two groups can be analysed with an independent sample t-test. In Table 9.2 the results of these analyses are shown.

From the results in Table 9.2 it can be seen that there is both a short-term and a long-term effect in favour of the therapy group, but that the long-term differences between the two groups are smaller than the short-term differences. This indicates that the short-term effect is stronger than the long-term effect. However, in Table 9.1 and in Figure 9.3 it was shown that at baseline there was a difference in systolic blood pressure between the therapy and the placebo groups. A better (but still simple) approach is therefore not to analyse the absolute systolic blood pressure values at $t = 2$ and $t = 3$, but to analyse the short-term and long-term differences in systolic blood pressure. In Chapter 8, the various possible ways in which to define change were extensively discussed, so that will not be repeated here. In this example the absolute differences were used. Obviously, the difference scores for the therapy and the placebo groups can be compared to each other with an independent sample t-test. Table 9.3 shows the results of these analyses.

The results presented in Table 9.3 show a totally different picture than the results in Table 9.2. The analysis of the differences between baseline and follow-up measurements did not show a beneficial effect of the therapy intervention compared with the placebo intervention. Although the differences for the therapy group were slightly greater than the differences for the placebo group in all comparisons, the independent sample t-test did not produce any significant difference. In conclusion, most of the assumed effect

Table 9.3. Mean values of the differences in systolic blood pressure between $t = 1$ and $t = 2$ and between $t = 1$ and $t = 3$; a comparison between therapy and placebo group and p-value derived from an independent sample t-test

	Therapy	Placebo	p-Value
Short-term difference[a]	3.38	0.64	0.189
Long-term difference[b]	4.23	3.13	0.616

[a] (Systolic blood pressure at $t = 1$) − (systolic blood pressure at $t = 2$).
[b] (Systolic blood pressure at $t = 1$) − (systolic blood pressure at $t = 3$).

of the therapy was already present at baseline. So this 'effect' could not be attributed to the therapy intervention.

9.2.3 Summary statistics

There are many summary statistics available with which to estimate the effect of an intervention in an experimental longitudinal study. In fact, the simple analyses carried out in Section 9.2.2 can also be considered as summary statistics. Depending on the research question to be addressed and the characteristics of the outcome variable, different summary statistics can be used. The general idea of a summary statistic is to express the longitudinal development of a particular outcome variable as one quantity. Therefore, the complicated longitudinal problem is reduced to a cross-sectional problem. To evaluate the effect of the intervention, the summary statistics of the groups under study are compared to each other. Table 9.4 gives a few examples of summary statistics.

One of the most frequently used summary statistics is the area under the curve (AUC). The AUC is calculated as shown in Equation (9.1):

$$\text{AUC} = \frac{1}{2} \sum_{t=1}^{T-1} (t_{t+1} - t_t)(Y_t + Y_{t+1}) \tag{9.1}$$

where AUC is the area under the curve, T is the number of measurements, and Y is the observation of the outcome variable at time t.

The unit of the AUC is the multiplication of the unit used for the outcome variable Y and the unit used for time. This is often rather difficult, and therefore the AUC is often divided by the total time period under consideration

Table 9.4. Examples of summary statistics which are frequently used in experimental studies

The mean of all follow-up measurements
The highest (or lowest) value during follow-up
The time needed to reach the highest value or a certain predefined level
Changes between baseline and follow-up levels
The area under the curve

Table 9.5. Area under the curve for systolic blood pressure between $t = 1$ and $t = 3$; a comparison between therapy and placebo group and p-value derived from an independent sample t-test

	Therapy	Placebo	p-Value
Area under the curve	246.51	259.23	0.007

in order to obtain a 'weighted' average level over the time period. When the AUC is used as a summary statistic, the AUC must first be calculated for each subject; this is then used as an outcome variable to evaluate the effect of the therapy under study. Again, this comparison is simple to carry out with an independent t-test. The result of the analysis is shown in Table 9.5.

From Table 9.5 it can be seen that a highly significant difference was found between the AUC values of the two groups. This will not directly indicate that the therapy intervention has an effect on the outcome variable. In the calculation, the difference in baseline value between the two groups is not taken into account. So, again, a difference in baseline value between groups can cause a difference in AUC.

When the time intervals are equally spaced (like in the example dataset), the AUC is comparable to the overall mean. The AUC becomes interesting when the time intervals in the longitudinal study are unequally spaced, because then the AUC reflects the 'weighted' average in a certain outcome variable over the total follow-up period.

9.2.4 MANOVA for repeated measurements

With the simple methods described in Section 9.2.2, separate analyses for short-term and long-term effects were performed. The purpose of summary

Output 9.1. Result of MANOVA for repeated measurements for systolic blood pressure (only the 'univariate' estimation procedure is presented)

AVERAGED Tests of Significance for SYSBP using UNIQUE sums of squares

Source of Variation	SS	DF	MS	F	Sig of F
WITHIN+RESIDUAL	55410.88	117	473.60		
GROUP	3122.56	1	3122.56	6.59	0.011

Source of Variation	SS	DF	MS	F	Sig of F
WITHIN+RESIDUAL	14854.68	234	63.48		
TIME	816.41	2	408.21	6.43	0.002
GROUP BY TIME	160.95	2	80.48	1.27	0.283

statistics, such as the AUC, is to summarize the total development of the outcome variable, in order to make simple cross-sectional analysis possible. Another way to analyse the total development of the outcome variable and to answer the question of whether the therapy has an effect on a certain outcome variable, is to use MANOVA for repeated measurements (see Chapter 3). Output 9.1 shows the result of the MANOVA for repeated measurements.

The output of the MANOVA for repeated measurements reveals that for systolic blood pressure there is an overall group effect ($F = 6.59$, $p = 0.011$), and an overall time effect ($F = 6.43$, $p = 0.002$), but no significant interaction between group and time ($F = 1.27$, $p = 0.283$). In particular, the information regarding the interaction is essential, because this indicates that the observed overall group effect does not change over time. This means that from the results of the MANOVA for repeated measurements it can be concluded that the two groups differ over time (a significant group effect), but that this difference is present along the whole longitudinal period, including the baseline measurement. So there is no 'real' therapy effect. From Figure 9.2 it can be seen that there is a decrease in systolic blood pressure over time. Because a decrease in systolic blood pressure is considered to be beneficial, a beneficial development is observed in both groups, which seems to be independent of the therapy intervention.

9.2.4.1 *MANOVA for repeated measurements corrected for the baseline value*

When the baseline values are different in the groups to be compared, it is often suggested that a MANOVA for repeated measurements should be

Output 9.2. Result of MANCOVA for repeated measurements for systolic blood pressure (only the 'univariate' estimation procedure is presented)

```
AVERAGED Tests of Significance for SYSBP using UNIQUE sums of squares
Source of Variation           SS       DF        MS         F     Sig of F
WITHIN+RESIDUAL           10836.93      116    93.422
GROUP                       539.47        1   539.47      5.77      0.018

Source of Variation           SS       DF        MS         F     Sig of F
WITHIN+RESIDUAL           12586.27      232    54.25
TIME                       1959.22        2   979.62     18.05      0.000
GROUP BY TIME               304.69        2   152.34      2.80      0.062
```

performed, correcting for the baseline value of the outcome variable. With this procedure the changes between the baseline measurement and the first follow-up measurement as well as the changes between the first and the second follow-up measurements are corrected for the baseline value.

It should be noted carefully that when this procedure (which is also known as multiple analysis of covariance, i.e. MANCOVA) is performed, the baseline value is both an outcome variable (i.e. to create the difference between the baseline value and the first follow-up measurement) and a covariate. In some software packages (such as SPSS) this is not possible, and therefore an exact copy of the baseline value must be added to the model. Output 9.2 shows the results of the MANCOVA.

From the results of Output 9.2 it can be seen that there is a significant therapy effect ($p = 0.018$). In the results obtained from the MANCOVA, the therapy by time interaction does not provide information about the 'direct' therapy effect. It provides information about whether the observed therapy effect is stronger at the beginning or at the end of the follow-up period. From the results it can be seen that the therapy by time interaction is almost significant ($p = 0.062$), but it is not clear during which part of the follow-up period the effect is the strongest. Therefore, a graphical representation of the MANCOVA results is needed (see Output 9.3). From Output 9.3 it can be seen that in the first part of the follow-up period, the therapy effect is the strongest. It should further be noted that the correction for baseline leads to equal starting points for both groups.

Output 9.3. Graphical representation of the results of the MANCOVA (—— placebo, – – – therapy)

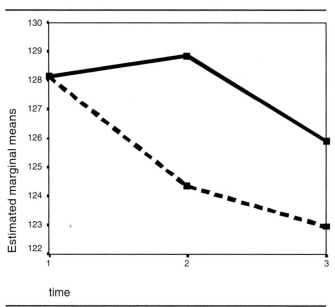

9.2.5 Sophisticated analysis

In the discussion on observational longitudinal studies (Chapter 4) it has already been mentioned that the questions answered by MANOVA for repeated measurements could also be answered by sophisticated methods (GEE analysis and random coefficient analysis). The advantage of the sophisticated methods is that all available data are included in the analysis, while with MANOVA for repeated measurements (and therefore also with MANCOVA) only those subjects with a complete dataset are included. In this example the MANOVA for repeated measurements (and the MANCOVA) was carried out for 118 patients, whereas with GEE analysis and random coefficient analysis all available data relating to all 152 patients can be used.

To analyse the effects of the therapy on systolic blood pressure, the following statistical model was first used (Equation (9.2)):

$$Y_{it} = \beta_0 + \beta_1 \times \text{therapy} + \beta_2 \times \text{time} + \varepsilon_{it} \tag{9.2}$$

where Y_{it} are observations for subject i at time t, β_0 is the intercept, β_1 is the regression coefficient for therapy versus placebo, β_2 is the regression coefficient for time, and ε_{it} is the 'error' for subject i at time t.

Output 9.4. Results of the GEE analysis with systolic blood pressure as outcome variable, and therapy and time as predictor variables

```
Linear Generalized Estimating Equations
Response: SYSBP    Corr: Exchangeable
Column  Name        Coeff   StErr   p-value
-------------------------------------------
     0  Constant  132.578   2.108     0.000
     2  TIME       -2.098   0.537     0.000
     3  THERAPY    -4.634   2.057     0.024
-------------------------------------------
n:152    s:14.326     #iter:13
Estimate of common correlation 0.654
```

First a GEE analysis was performed, in which an exchangeable correlation structure was chosen (for a detailed discussion on different correlation structures, see Section 4.5.2). Output 9.4 shows the result of this GEE analysis. From Output 9.4 it can be seen that therapy has a significant negative association with the development of systolic blood pressure ($\beta = -4.634$, standard error 2.057, $p = 0.024$). This does not mean that the therapy has an effect on systolic blood pressure, because it is possible that the association was already present at baseline. In fact, the analysis performed is only suitable in a situation in which the baseline values of the outcome variable are equal for the therapy group and the placebo group. To analyse the 'real' therapy effect, a second GEE analysis has to be carried out in which the therapy by time interaction is also added to the model (Equation (9.3)).

$$Y_{it} = \beta_0 + \beta_1 \times \text{therapy} + \beta_2 \times \text{time} + \beta_3 \times \text{therapy} \times \text{time} + \varepsilon_{it} \qquad (9.3)$$

where Y_{it} are observations for subject i at time t, β_0 is the intercept, β_1 is the regression coefficient for therapy versus placebo, β_2 is the regression coefficient for time, β_3 is the regression coefficient for the therapy by time interaction, and ε_{it} is the 'error' for subject i at time t.

The results of this analysis are shown in Output 9.5.

Output 9.5. Results of the GEE analysis with systolic blood pressure as outcome variable and therapy, time and the interaction between therapy and time as predictor variables

```
Linear Generalized Estimating Equations
Response: SYSBP              Corr: Exchangeable
Column   Name                Coeff   StErr   p-value
----------------------------------------------------
     0   Constant           132.214  2.462    0.000
     2   TIME                -1.912  0.747    0.010
     3   THERAPY             -3.894  3.142    0.215
     4   THERAPY*TIME        -0.378  1.074    0.725
----------------------------------------------------
n:152    s:14.343   #iter:10
Estimate of common correlation 0.654
```

When an interaction term is added to the analysis, the most interesting part is the significance level of the interaction term, which is 0.725 in this example. This interaction is not close to significance, so we can conclude that there is a negative association between therapy and systolic blood pressure

Output 9.6. Results of the random coefficient analysis with systolic blood pressure as outcome variable *Y*, and therapy and time as predictor variables; a random intercept and a random slope with time are considered

```
log likelihood = -1596.9878
-----------------------------------------------------------------------------
  sysbp        Coeff   Std. Err.      z    P > |z|   [95% Conf.    Interval]
-----------------------------------------------------------------------------
therapy    -4.878309  2.037021   -2.395   0.017   -8.870797   -0.8858217
   time    -2.081433  0.5364209  -3.880   0.000   -3.132799   -1.030068
  _cons   132.5799    1.824256   72.676   0.000   129.0045    136.1554
-----------------------------------------------------------------------------

Variance at level 1
-----------------------------------------------------------------------------
63.856006   (7.3923457)

Variances and covariances of random effects
-----------------------------------------------------------------------------
***level 2 (id)

  var(1): 206.76445   (44.841986)
cov(1,2): -22.372747 (14.005004)   cor(1,2): -0.69024558
  var(2):   5.0810734 (5.6104568)
```

(see Output 9.2), but that this association does not change over time. So (probably) the difference is already present at baseline, a finding which was already observed in earlier analysis. It is important to notice that when an interaction term is added to the model, the regression coefficients (and the significance levels) of the separate variables can only be interpreted in combination with the regression coefficients of the interaction term. As expected, when a random coefficient analysis was applied, the results were comparable. Outputs 9.6 and 9.7 present the results of the random coefficient analysis.

Output 9.7. Results of the random coefficient analysis with systolic blood pressure as outcome variable, and therapy, time and the interaction between therapy and time as predictor variables; a random intercept and a random slope with time are considered

```
log likelihood = -1596.9146
--------------------------------------------------------------------
    sysbp      Coeff   Std. Err.     z    P > |z|  [95% Conf.   Interval]
--------------------------------------------------------------------
  therapy  -3.961371   3.143711   -1.260   0.208  -10.12293    2.200189
     time  -1.879885  0.7508875   -2.504   0.012   -3.351597  -0.4081722
  ther*tim -0.4096528  1.070124   -0.383   0.702   -2.507058   1.687752
    _cons  132.1346    2.162306   61.108   0.000   127.8966   136.3726
--------------------------------------------------------------------

Variance at level 1
--------------------------------------------------------------------
63.925841   (7.3772168)

Variances and covariances of random effects
--------------------------------------------------------------------
***level 2 (id)

  var(1): 206.38405   (44.695857)
cov(1,2): -22.203339 (13.923335) cor(1,2): -0.69271147
  var(2):   4.9780094 (5.570582)
```

In addition to the use of an interaction term, there is an alternative approach to the analysis of data in an experimental longitudinal study in which the baseline values of a particular outcome variable are different. In this approach, which is known as analysis of covariance, the values of an outcome variable Y at $t = 2$ and $t = 3$ are related to therapy, correcting for the baseline value of Y at $t = 1$ (Equation (9.4)).

$$Y_{it} = \beta_0 + \beta_1 \times \text{therapy} + \beta_2 \times \text{time} + \beta_3 \, Y_{t1} + \varepsilon_{it} \qquad (9.4)$$

where Y_{it} are observations for subject i at time t, β_0 is the intercept, β_1 is the regression coefficient for therapy versus placebo, β_2 is the regression coefficient for time, β_3 is the regression coefficient for the baseline value of Y, and ε_{it} is the 'error' for subject i at time t.

This model looks similar to the autoregression model which was described in Chapter 5 (Section 5.2.3), but it is slightly different. In the autoregression model, a correction was made for the value of the outcome variable at $t = t - 1$. In the analysis of covariance, a correction is made for the baseline value of the outcome variable (see also Section 8.2). Output 9.8 shows the results of the GEE analysis (based on Equation (9.4)) for systolic blood pressure. Surprisingly, in the GEE analysis a significant therapy effect was found. For therapy, a regression coefficient of -3.68 was found, which indicates that the therapy group has a 3.68 mmHg lower systolic blood pressure than the placebo group. Comparable results were found with random coefficient analysis (see Output 9.9).

Output 9.8. Results of the GEE analysis with systolic blood pressure as outcome variable, and therapy, time and the baseline value of systolic blood pressure as predictor variables

```
Linear Generalized Estimating Equations
Response: SYSBP     Corr: Exchangeable
Column    Name          Coeff     StErr      p-value
------------------------------------------------------
    0     Constant     51.208    10.221      0.000
    2     THERAPY      -3.684     1.534      0.016
    3     TIME         -1.915     1.037      0.065
    5     SYSBPT1       0.615     0.080      0.000
------------------------------------------------------
n:130     s:10.48      #iter:24
Estimate of common correlation 0.352
```

The results derived from the sophisticated analysis are comparable to the results obtained from the MANOVA and MANCOVA comparison. In the analysis with interaction terms, no significant difference was found between the therapy group and the placebo group, while in the analysis of covariance a significant therapy effect was observed. The difference between a longitudinal

Output 9.9. Results of a random coefficient analysis with systolic blood pressure as outcome variable, and therapy, time and the baseline value of systolic blood pressure as predictor variables

```
log likelihood = -927.31482
------------------------------------------------------------------------
   sysbp       Coeff    Std. Err.      z      P > |z|   [95% Conf.   Interval]
------------------------------------------------------------------------
  therapy   -3.665562   1.576142    -2.326    0.020    -6.754744   -0.5763806
     time   -1.932226   1.036378    -1.864    0.062    -3.963489    0.099038
  sysbpt1    0.6126458  0.0520755   11.765    0.000     0.5105797   0.714712
    _cons   51.47565    7.058234     7.293    0.000    37.64177    65.30953
------------------------------------------------------------------------

Variance at level 1
------------------------------------------------------------------------
63.276222    (8.7697865)
Variances and covariances of random effects
------------------------------------------------------------------------
***level 2 (id)

 var(1):  59.642216   (36.495775)
cov(1,2): -8.3496959  (14.099664) cor(1,2): -0.50792301
 var(2):   4.530976   (3.27834)
```

analysis correcting for the baseline value and the longitudinal analysis with an interaction term is that in the latter basically the difference between Y at $t = 1$ and Y at $t = 2$ and the difference between Y at $t = 2$ and Y at $t = 3$ are combined in one analysis, while in the analysis of covariance (i.e. correcting for the baseline values) the difference between Y at $t = 1$ and Y at $t = 2$ and the difference between Y at $t = 1$ and Y at $t = 3$ are analysed simultaneously. A difference in results between the two methods probably indicates that there is a small but consistent therapy effect, or that the therapy effect mostly occurs at the beginning of the follow-up period. This (small) effect is not detected by the analysis with an interaction term, but is detected by the approach correcting for the baseline value. In fact, the correction for baseline over-estimates the therapy effect, because the short-term effect is doubled in the estimation of the overall therapy effect. This situation is illustrated in Figure 9.4. A possible solution for this over-estimation is the use of an autoregressive model (see Section 5.2.3) instead of a correction for the baseline value.

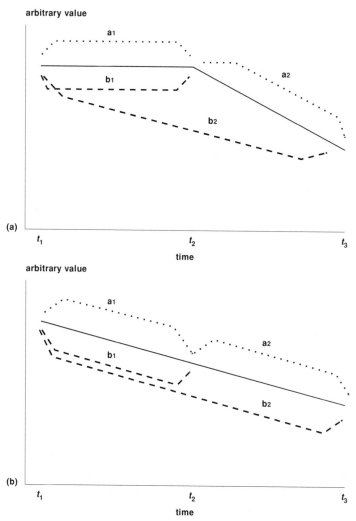

Figure 9.4. Illustration of the difference between two approaches that can be used in the analysis of an experimental longitudinal study. The effects a1 and a2 are detected by the analysis with an interaction term (Equation (9.3)), while the effects b1 and b2 are detected by the longitudinal analysis, correcting for the baseline value (Equation (9.4)). For the situation in (a), the two methods will show comparable results (a1 = b1 and a2 = b2). For the situation shown in (b), the longitudinal analysis, correcting for baseline, will detect a stronger decline than the analysis with an interaction term (a1 = b1 and a2 < b2). The situation in (c) will produce the same result as (b) (i.e. a1 = b1 and a2 < b2) (——— outcome variable).

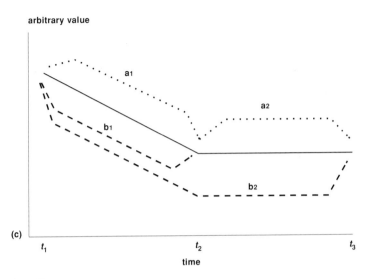

Figure 9.4. (*cont.*)

9.3 Example with a dichotomous outcome variable

9.3.1 Introduction

The example of an experimental study with a dichotomous outcome variable uses a dataset from a hypothetical study in which a new drug is tested on patients with a stomach ulcer. Treatment duration is 1 month, and patients are seen at three follow-up visits. The first follow-up visit is directly at the end of the intervention period (after 1 month) and the two long-term follow-up visits 6 and 12 months, respectively, after the start of the intervention. In this randomized controlled trial (RCT), the intervention (i.e. the new drug) is compared to a placebo, and 60 patients were included in each of the two groups. In the follow-up period of 1 year, there was no loss to follow-up, and therefore no missing data. Figure 9.5 shows the proportion of patients who had fully recovered at the different follow-up measurements.

9.3.2 Simple analysis

The classical way to analyse the results of such an RCT is to analyse the difference in proportion of patients experiencing full recovery between the intervention and the placebo group at each of the three follow-up measurements,

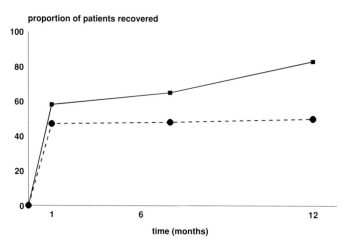

Figure 9.5. The proportion of patients recovered in an RCT to investigate the effect of an intervention (i.e. a new drug) (■ —— intervention, ● – – – placebo).

by simply applying a χ^2 test. Furthermore, at each of the follow-up measurements, the effect of the intervention can be estimated by calculating the relative risk (and corresponding 95% confidence interval). The relative risk is defined as the proportion of subjects recovered in the intervention group, divided by the proportion of subjects recovered in the placebo group. The results are summarized in Table 9.6.

From the results in Table 9.6 it can be seen that during the intervention period of 1 month both the intervention group and the placebo group show quite a high proportion of patients who recover, and although in the intervention group this proportion is slightly higher, the difference is not statistically significant ($p = 0.20$). After the intervention period, in both groups there is an increase in the number of patients who recovered, but in the intervention group this increase is more pronounced, which results in a significant difference between the intervention group and the placebo group after 1 year of follow-up.

9.3.3 Sophisticated analysis

Although this RCT is a longitudinal study, up to now only simple cross-sectional analyses have been performed. After these simple analyses, a sophisticated longitudinal analysis can be carried out to investigate the difference

Table 9.6. Results of an RCT to investigate the effect of an intervention, i.e. the number of patients recovered, the 'relative risks' and 95% confidence intervals (in parentheses) for the intervention group and the corresponding p-values at each of the follow-up measurements

	Recovery after 1 month		Recovery after 6 months		Recovery after 12 months	
	Yes	No	Yes	No	Yes	No
Intervention	35	25	39	21	60	10
Placebo	28	32	29	31	30	30
Relative risk	1.28 (0.87–1.88)		1.48 (0.97–2.53)		3.00 (1.61–5.58)	
p-Value	0.20		0.07		< 0.01	

in the total development of recovery between the intervention and placebo groups over the follow-up period of 1 year. A logistic GEE analysis was carried out to illustrate the possibilities and limitations of the sophisticated longitudinal analysis. In this example, only a GEE analysis will be considered, and not a random coefficient analysis, because the main interest lies in the 'population average' estimates (for a detailed discussion regarding the differences between GEE analysis and random coefficient analysis with dichotomous outcome variables, see Section 6.2.5). The first thing that should be realized is that as a result of a logistic GEE analysis, odds ratios can be calculated. Odds ratios can be interpreted as relative risks, but they are not the same. Owing to the mathematical background of the odds ratios and relative risks, the odds ratios are always an over-estimation of the 'real' relative risk. This over-estimation becomes stronger as the proportion of 'cases' (i.e. recovered patients) increases. To illustrate this, the odds ratios for intervention versus placebo were calculated at each of the follow-up measurements (see Table 9.7).

From the results in Table 9.7 it can be seen that the calculated odds ratios are an over-estimation of the 'real' relative risks, and that the confidence intervals are wider, but that the significance levels are the same. So, when a logistic GEE analysis is carried out, one must realize that the results (i.e. odds ratios) obtained from such an analysis have to be interpreted with caution, and cannot be directly interpreted as relative risks.

Output 9.10 presents the results of the GEE analysis (assuming an exchangeable correlation structure), in which the following research question

Table 9.7. Comparison between relative risks and odds ratios, including 95% confidence intervals (in parentheses) and *p*-values as a result of an RCT to investigate the effect of an intervention

	1 month	6 months	12 months
Relative risk	1.28 (0.87–1.88)	1.48 (0.97–2.53)	3.00 (1.61–5.58)
p-Value	0.20	0.07	< 0.01
Odds ratio	1.60 (0.78–3.29)	1.99 (0.95–4.13)	5.00 (2.14–11.66)
p-Value	0.20	0.07	< 0.01

Output 9.10. Results of the GEE analysis to compare an intervention with a placebo with regard to recovery (a dichotomous outcome variable) measured over a period of one year

```
Binomial Generalized Estimating Equations
Response: RECOV     Corr: Exchangeable
Column   Name        Coeff   StErr   p-value   Odds    95%      CI
--------------------------------------------------------------------
     0   Constant   -1.472   0.192    0.000
     2   TIME        0.176   0.020    0.000    1.192   1.147    1.239
     3   INTERV      0.742   0.251    0.003    2.100   1.284    3.435
--------------------------------------------------------------------
n:120   s:0.999   #iter:10
Estimate of common correlation 0.149
```

was answered: 'What is the effect of the intervention (compared to the placebo) on recovery over a period of 1 year?' In the analysis firstly a linear relationship with time is modelled (i.e. time is coded as 0, 1, 6 and 12).

From Output 9.10 it can be seen that the intervention is highly successful over the total follow-up period (i.e. odds ratio 2.10, 95% confidence interval 1.28 to 3.44). As all patients were ill at baseline (by definition), there are no differences at baseline, so it is useless to correct for baseline values. It is also not really interesting to investigate the interaction between the intervention and time, because the main effect of the intervention already implies that the intervention is successful over the 1-year follow-up period. This is in contrast with the example presented in Section 9.2, in which there was a continuous outcome variable and the baseline values of the intervention and the placebo group differed. In that case the interaction between time and the intervention was necessary to evaluate the effect of the intervention (or a correction for the baseline value would have to be performed).

In the present example, a possible significant interaction between the intervention and time will give information about whether the effect of the intervention is stronger at the beginning of the follow-up period or stronger at the end of the follow-up period. Output 9.11 shows the results of the GEE analysis with the interaction between the intervention and time included in the model. From Output 9.11 it can be seen that there is a significant interaction between the intervention and time ($p = 0.003$). The sign of the regression coefficient of the interaction term is positive, which indicates that the effect of the intervention is stronger at the end of the follow-up period. This effect was already noticed in the separate analyses at each of the follow-up measurements (see Table 9.6)

Output 9.11. Results of the GEE analysis to compare an intervention with a placebo with regard to recovery (a dichotomous outcome variable) measured over a period of one year, with the interaction between time and intervention

```
Binomial Generalized Estimating Equations
Response: RECOV     Corr: Exchangeable
Column  Name        Coeff  StErr  p-value   Odds    95%     CI
-----------------------------------------------------------------
     0  Constant   -1.158  0.170   0.000
     2  TIME        0.119  0.025   0.000   1.126   1.072   1.184
     3  INTERV      0.164  0.231   0.479   1.178   0.748   1.854
     4  INT*TIME    0.129  0.043   0.003   1.137   1.046   1.237
-----------------------------------------------------------------
n:120   s:1.006   #iter:10
Estimate of common correlation 0.166
```

One must realize, however, that in the GEE models time is coded as 0, 1, 6 and 12. So, in the analysis a linear development in time is assumed. From Figure 9.4 it can be seen that the relationship with time is far from linear, so a second GEE analysis was performed, assuming a quadratic relationship with time. Output 9.12 shows the results of this analysis.

From Output 9.12 it can be seen that not only the linear component, but also the quadratic component of the relationship between the outcome

Output 9.12. Results of the GEE analysis to compare an intervention with a placebo with regard to recovery (a dichotomous outcome variable), measured over a period of one year, assuming a quadratic relationship with time

```
Binomial Generalized Estimating Equations
Response: RECOV      Corr: Exchangeable
Column   Name        Coeff   StErr   p-value    Odds     95%       CI
-----------------------------------------------------------------------
    0   Constant    -1.884   0.208    0.000
    2   TIME         0.523   0.060    0.000    1.688    1.501    1.898
    3   INTERV       0.798   0.268    0.003    2.221    1.313    3.756
    5   TIME**2     -0.029   0.005    0.000    0.972    0.936    0.980
-----------------------------------------------------------------------
n:120   s:0.992   #iter:12
Estimate of common correlation 0.161
```

variable and time is highly significant ($p < 0.001$). It is therefore better to model a quadratic development in time, in order to obtain a more valid estimate of the effect of the intervention. Calculated with this model, the effect of the intervention expressed as an odds ratio is 2.22 (95% confidence interval 1.31 to 3.76). Therefore, with the intervention drug, a patient is 2.22 times more likely to recover than with a placebo, calculated over a follow-up period of 1 year. In the model that only included a linear relationship with time, the odds ratio of the intervention (versus placebo) was 2.10 (95% confidence interval 1.28 to 3.44). Again, it should be noted that the odds ratios are an over-estimation of the 'real' relative risks.

9.4 Comments

The analyses discussed for both the continuous and dichotomous outcome variables in experimental studies were limited to 'crude' analyses, in such a way that no confounders (apart from the value of the outcome variable at baseline in the example of a continuous outcome variable) and/or effect modifiers (apart from the interaction between therapy/intervention and time in both examples) have been discussed. Potential effect modifiers can be interesting if one wishes to investigate whether the intervention effect is different for sub-groups of the population under study. The way confounders and effect modifiers are treated in longitudinal data analysis is, however, exactly the same as in simple cross-sectional regression analysis. The construction of prognostic models with variables measured at baseline, which is quite popular in clinical epidemiology these days, is also the same as in cross-sectional analysis.

In the examples of the sophisticated analyses, time was modelled as a continuous variable, i.e. either as a linear function or a quadratic function. However, as in the case of observational longitudinal studies when there is no linear relationship between the outcome variable and time, time can also be modelled as a categorical variable (see Section 4.8).

In both examples discussed in this chapter, the first analyses performed were simple cross-sectional analyses. In fact, it is recommended that statistical analysis to evaluate the effect of an intervention should always start with a simple analysis. This not only provides insight into the data, but can also provide (important) information regarding the effect of the intervention. It should also be noted that, although the simple techniques and summary statistics are somewhat limited, the interpretation of the results is often easy, and their use in clinical practice is therefore very popular. In general, to answer many research questions the simple techniques and summary statistics are quite adequate, and there is no real need to use the sophisticated techniques. Moreover, the results of the sophisticated techniques are (sometimes) difficult to interpret. However, when the number of repeated measurements differs between subjects, and/or when there are many missing observations, it is (highly) recommended that the more sophisticated statistical analyses should be applied.

Missing data in longitudinal studies

10.1 Introduction

One of the main methodological problems in longitudinal studies is missing data or attrition, i.e. the (unpleasant) situation when not all N subjects have data on all T measurements. When subjects have missing data at the end of a longitudinal study they are often referred to as **drop-outs**. It is, however, also possible that subjects miss one particular measurement, and then return to the study at the next follow-up. This type of missing data is often referred to as **intermittent** missing data (Figure 10.1). It should be noted that, in practice, drop-outs and intermittent missing data usually occur together.

In the statistical literature a distinction is made between three types of missing data: (1) missing completely at random (MCAR: missing, independent of both unobserved and observed data), (2) missing at random (MAR: missing, dependent on observed data, but not on unobserved data, or, in other words, given the observed data, the unobserved data are random), and (3) missing not at random (MNAR: missing, dependent on unobserved data) (Little and Rubin, 1987). Missing at random usually occurs when data are missing by design. An illustrative example is the Longitudinal Aging Study Amsterdam (Deeg and Westendorp-de Serière, 1994). In this observational longitudinal study, a large cohort of elderly subjects was screened for the clinical existence of depression. Because the number of non-depressed subjects was much greater than the number of depressed subjects, a random sample of non-depressed subjects was selected for the follow-up, in combination with the total group of depressed subjects. So, given the fact that the subjects were not depressed, the data were missing at random (see Figure 10.2).

Although the above-mentioned distinction between the three different types of missing data is important, it is rather theoretical. For a correct

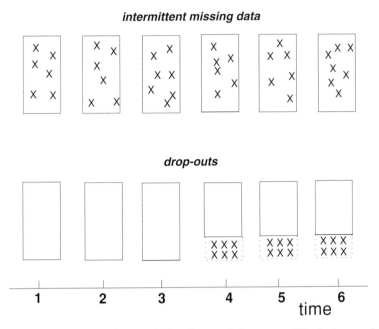

Figure 10.1. Illustration of intermittent missing data and drop-outs (X indicates a missing data point).

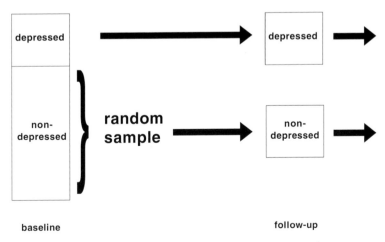

Figure 10.2. An illustration of data missing by design, i.e. missing at random.

interpretation of the results of longitudinal data analysis, two issues must be considered. First of all, it is important to investigate whether or not missing data on the outcome variable Y at a certain time-point are dependent on the values of the outcome variable observed one (or more) time-point(s) earlier. In other words, it is important to investigate whether or not missing data depend on earlier observations. Secondly, it is important to determine whether or not certain predictor variables are related to the occurrence of missing data. For example, 'are males more likely to have missing data than females?' In general, it is preferable to make a distinction between 'ignorable' missing data (i.e. missing, **not dependent** on earlier observations and predictor variables) and 'non-ignorable' or 'informative' missing data (i.e. missing, **dependent** on earlier observations or predictor variables).

10.2 Ignorable or informative missing data?

Although there is an abundance of statistical literature describing (complicated) methods that can be used to investigate whether or not one is dealing with ignorable or informative missing data in a longitudinal study (see, for instance, Diggle, 1989; Ridout, 1991; Diggle et al., 1994), it is basically quite easy to investigate this matter. It can be done by comparing the group of subjects with data at $t = t$ with the group of subjects with missing data at $t = t$. First of all, this comparison can concern the particular outcome variable of interest measured at $t = t - 1$. Depending on the distribution of that particular variable, an independent sample t-test (for continuous variables) or a χ^2 test (for dichotomous and categorical outcome variables) can be carried out. Secondly, the influence of certain predictor variables on the occurrence of missing data can be investigated. This can be done by means of a (simple) logistic regression analysis, with missing or non-missing at each of the repeated measurements as a dichotomous outcome variable.

Up to now, a distinction has been made between missing data dependent on earlier values of the outcome variable Y and missing data dependent on values of possible predictor variables. Of course, this distinction is not really necessary, because in practice they both occur together and can both be investigated with logistic regression analysis, with both the earlier value of the outcome variable and the values of the predictor variables as possible determinants for why the data are missing. It should be noted that the distinction is made purely for educational purposes.

When there are only a few (repeated) measurements, and when the amount of missing data at each of the (repeated) measurements is rather high, the above-mentioned procedures are highly suitable to investigate whether one is dealing with ignorable or informative missing data. However, when the amount of missing data at a particular measurement is rather low, the power to detect differences between the subjects with data and the subjects without data at a particular time-point can be too low. Although the possible significance of the differences is not the most important issue in determining whether or not the pattern of missing data is ignorable or informative, it can be problematic to interpret the observed differences correctly. Therefore, the information about missing data at different time-points can be combined (Diggle, 1989; Ridout, 1991; Diggle et al., 1994). However, the statistical techniques involved are seldom used in practice.

10.3 Example

10.3.1 Generating datasets with missing data

The dataset used to illustrate the influence of missing data on the results of statistical analysis is the same example dataset which has been used throughout this book (see Section 1.4). All incomplete datasets were derived from the full dataset, and at each time-point only the outcome variable Y is assumed to be missing. In this example, a situation with both drop-outs and intermittent missing data will be considered.

In the datasets with drop-outs the first three measurements were completed by all subjects, but from the fourth measurements onwards data on 25% of the individuals were missing. The missing data were considered to be random (i.e. ignorable missing data) and dependent on the value of the outcome variable Y at the third measurement (i.e. informative missing data), i.e. data on the subjects with the highest values for the outcome variable Y at $t = 3$ were assumed to be missing at $t = 4$, $t = 5$ and $t = 6$.

In the datasets with intermittent missing data, at each repeated measurement (including the initial measurement at $t = 1$) 25% of the data were missing. Again this was assumed to be at random (i.e. ignorable missing data) or dependent on the observed data (i.e. informative missing data), i.e. data on the subjects with the highest values for the outcome variable Y at $t = t$ were assumed to be missing at $t = t + 1$. In this example dataset with informative missing data, a full dataset at $t = 1$ was considered.

Table 10.1. Results of independent sample *t*-tests to compare the drop-outs after $t = 3$ with the non-drop-outs, according to the value of the outcome variable Y at $t = 3$

	N	Mean(Y_{t1})	t-Value	Degrees of freedom	p-Value
Ignorable					
Missing	33	4.24	0.25	145	0.807
Not missing	114	4.27			
Informative					
Missing	39	5.20	15.91	145	<0.001
Not missing	108	3.93			

10.3.2 Analysis of determinants for missing data

As has been mentioned in the introduction of this chapter, it is important to investigate whether or not the missing data are dependent either on earlier values of the outcome variable or on the values of certain predictor variables. This knowledge can have important implications for the interpretation of the results of a longitudinal study.

It is quite simple to investigate whether the missing data are dependent on values of the outcome variable Y one time-point earlier. This can be done by comparing the subjects with data at $t = t$ with the subjects with missing data at $t = t$. The comparison is then performed on the value of the outcome variable at $t = t - 1$. The difference between the two groups can be tested with an independent sample *t*-test. In this example, only the dataset with drop-outs will be used for illustration, but comparable analyses can be performed for the dataset with intermittent missing data.

In Table 10.1, the results of the independent sample *t*-tests are given for the dataset with drop-outs. Owing to the structure of the missing data, the type of missing data at $t = 4$ is analysed. So the subjects with missing data at $t = 4$ are compared with the subjects with data at $t = 4$, according to the value of the outcome variable Y at $t = 3$.

Because the missing datasets are forced to be either ignorable or informative, the results are as expected. Considerable differences were found in the outcome variable Y at $t = 3$ between the subjects with data and the subjects without data at $t = 4$, when the missing data were forced to be informative. No significant differences were found in the dataset with ignorable missing

Table 10.2. Regression coefficients and p-values of logistic regression analyses to investigate possible determinants (measured at $t = 3$) for drop-out after $t = 3$

	X_1	X_2	X_3	X_4
Ignorable	1.36 ($p = 0.26$)	0.17 ($p = 0.17$)	0.59 ($p = 0.54$)	-0.06 ($p = 0.91$)
Informative	0.16 ($p = 0.89$)	0.58 ($p < 0.01$)	-0.21 ($p = 0.71$)	0.04 ($p = 0.94$)

data. The independent sample t-test is only performed to determine whether the missing data are dependent on the outcome variable one time-point earlier. It is also of interest to analyse other possible determinants of the missing data. Information about these determinants can be important for correct interpretation of the results of a longitudinal study with missing data. A logistic regression analysis was subsequently performed, with missing at $t = 4$ and not missing at $t = 4$ as the dichotomous outcome variable. The values of the four predictor variables in the example dataset (X_1 to X_4) at $t = 3$ were analysed as potential determinants for the missing data. In Table 10.2 the results of the logistic regression analyses are summarized.

From the results presented in Table 10.2 it can be seen that it is only in the dataset with informative missing data that subjects with high values of X_2 at $t = 3$ seem to have a higher 'chance' of having missing data at $t = 4$. This is not really surprising, because from earlier analyses of the example dataset it is already known that X_2 and Y are associated with each other. So, when missing data are found to be dependent on the value of Y one measurement earlier, it can be expected that this is also the case for X_2.

The analyses described in this section illustrate how to investigate possible determinants of the missing data. In the example datasets these analyses were not really interesting, because the datasets with missing data were forced to be either informative or ignorable. However, in practice it is necessary to investigate both issues, because interpretation of the results highly depends on the 'nature' of the missing data.

10.4 Analysis performed on datasets with missing data

In the foregoing paragraphs it was stressed that it is important to investigate whether one is dealing with ignorable or informative missing data. First of all, it is important to invoke a correct interpretation of the results of the statistical analysis performed on the 'incomplete' dataset. Secondly, it is also important because the sophisticated statistical techniques (i.e. GEE analysis and random coefficient analysis) differ in the way in which they treat missing data. In fact, in the literature it is often argued that one of the most important differences between GEE analysis and random coefficient analysis is found in the analysis of datasets with missing data. The difference is that with GEE analysis the missing data are assumed to be missing completely at random (MCAR), and that in random coefficient analysis the missing data are assumed to be missing at random (MAR) (Little, 1995; Albert, 1999; Omar et al., 1999). When GEE analysis is performed on an incomplete dataset with informative missing data, the calculation of the working correlation structure is biased, and therefore the calculation of the regression coefficients is also assumed to be biased. However, from the literature it is not clear how important this bias really is.

It is therefore interesting to analyse the missing datasets with both GEE analysis and random coefficient analysis, and to compare the results. Furthermore, it was mentioned earlier that one of the advantages of both GEE analysis and random coefficient analysis compared, for instance, to MANOVA for repeated measurements, is that with the sophisticated techniques all longitudinal data are included, while in the (traditional) MANOVA for repeated measurements only the subjects with complete data are included in the analysis. Therefore, in the example (Section 10.4.1) all analyses (i.e. MANOVA, GEE analysis and random coefficient analysis) will be performed on the datasets with missing data that were described in Section 10.3.1.

10.4.1 Example

Table 10.3 shows the results of MANOVA for repeated measurements for the complete dataset and the datasets with missing data. With MANOVA for repeated measurements, the overall difference between two groups (indicated by X_4, i.e. males and females), the overall development in time, and the possible difference in development over time between the two groups (indicated by the time by X_4 interaction) were investigated. For both the within-subject effects (i.e. the effects involving time), and the between-subjects effect (i.e. the overall group difference), explained variances were calculated (see Chapter 3).

The most important difference between the results of the MANOVA on incomplete datasets and the results of the MANOVA on a complete dataset

Table 10.3. Explained variances and *p*-values derived from a MANOVA for repeated measurements performed on a complete dataset and several incomplete datasets

	X_4	Time	Time by X_4
Complete dataset	0.04 ($p = 0.01$)	0.42 ($p < 0.01$)	0.05 ($p < 0.01$)
Drop-outs			
Ignorable	0.03 ($p = 0.05$)	0.43 ($p < 0.01$)	0.05 ($p < 0.01$)
Informative	0.01 ($p = 0.23$)	0.48 ($p < 0.01$)	0.09 ($p < 0.01$)
Intermittent missing data			
Ignorable	0.06 ($p = 0.29$)	0.40 ($p < 0.01$)	0.01 ($p = 0.01$)
Informative	0.02 ($p = 0.29$)	0.51 ($p < 0.01$)	0.01 ($p < 0.01$)

are observed for the between-subjects effect of X_4. This is not reflected in a difference in explained variance, but in the *p*-values. The fact that the *p*-values are much higher in the datasets with missing data is due to the fact that with MANOVA for repeated measurements **only** the subjects with complete data are included in the analysis. So, particularly in the dataset with intermittent missing data, the power of the analysis is highly reduced. From the results it can be seen that there seems to be no influence of the type of missing data. This is not really surprising, because in the dataset with informative missing data, these missing data were forced to be dependent on earlier observations of the outcome variable Y, and from Table 10.2 it was already known that the missing data were independent of the value of X_4.

Table 10.4 shows the results of the GEE analysis, and Table 10.5 shows the results of the random coefficient analysis. With both techniques the longitudinal relationship between outcome variable Y and the four predictor variables X_1 to X_4 and time was analysed. The regression coefficients and standard errors calculated with the different methods used to analyse the incomplete datasets are only slightly different to those obtained from the analysis of the complete dataset. Furthermore, the differences found in the datasets with informative missing data are no greater than the differences found in the datasets with ignorable missing data. So, in this particular situation, both GEE analysis and random coefficient analysis are 'valid' in research situations with missing data, even when the missing data are (highly)

Table 10.4. Regression coefficients and standard errors (in parentheses) derived from a GEE analysis[a] performed on a complete dataset and several incomplete datasets to investigate the (longitudinal) relationship between outcome variable Y and several predictor variables

	X_1	X_2	X_3	X_4	Time
Complete dataset	−0.02 (0.27)	0.11 (0.02)	−0.11 (0.06)	0.10 (0.12)	0.11 (0.01)
Drop-outs					
Ignorable	0.05 (0.26)	0.14 (0.02)	−0.10 (0.07)	0.05 (0.13)	0.10 (0.02)
Informative	0.05 (0.27)	0.15 (0.03)	−0.07 (0.07)	0.05 (0.13)	0.07 (0.01)
Intermittent missing data					
Ignorable	0.06 (0.27)	0.13 (0.02)	−0.10 (0.07)	0.09 (0.14)	0.09 (0.02)
Informative	0.07 (0.29)	0.13 (0.02)	−0.05 (0.07)	0.08 (0.13)	0.09 (0.01)

[a] GEE analysis with an exchangeable correlation structure.

Table 10.5. Regression coefficients and standard errors (in parentheses) derived from a random coefficient analysis[a] performed on a complete dataset and several incomplete datasets to investigate the (longitudinal) relationship between outcome variable Y and several predictor variables

	X_1	X_2	X_3	X_4	Time
Complete dataset	0.02 (0.27)	0.11 (0.02)	−0.12 (0.06)	0.04 (0.12)	0.11 (0.01)
Drop-outs					
Ignorable	0.06 (0.27)	0.14 (0.02)	−0.11 (0.06)	0.02 (0.12)	0.10 (0.01)
Informative	0.05 (0.27)	0.15 (0.02)	−0.08 (0.06)	0.05 (0.12)	0.07 (0.01)
Intermittent missing data					
Ignorable	0.03 (0.28)	0.13 (0.02)	−0.05 (0.07)	0.01 (0.12)	0.09 (0.01)
Informative	0.05 (0.28)	0.13 (0.02)	−0.06 (0.06)	0.04 (0.12)	0.09 (0.01)

[a] Random coefficient analysis with both a random intercept and a random slope with time.

informative. In other words, for a continuous outcome variable the differences between GEE analysis and random coefficient analysis with incomplete datasets are not as obvious as is often suggested. The results are, again, an indication that the assumed differences between the two techniques are more theoretical than practical.

Table 10.6. Regression coefficients and standard errors (in parentheses) derived from a GEE analysis[a] performed on a complete dataset and several incomplete datasets to investigate the (longitudinal) relationship between the dichotomous outcome variable Y and several predictor variables

	X_1	X_2	X_3	X_4	Time
Complete dataset	0.22 (0.77)	0.34 (0.06)	−0.15 (0.18)	0.08 (0.34)	−0.08 (0.04)
Drop-outs					
Ignorable	0.48 (0.79)	0.40 (0.02)	−0.02 (0.34)	−0.04 (0.19)	−0.08 (0.04)
Informative	0.37 (0.76)	0.40 (0.07)	0.03 (0.33)	−0.05 (0.22)	−0.12 (0.04)
Intermittent missing data					
Ignorable	0.17 (0.79)	0.39 (0.07)	−0.09 (0.19)	0.05 (0.39)	−0.09 (0.04)
Informative	0.42 (0.81)	0.40 (0.07)	0.03 (0.19)	0.03 (0.38)	−0.09 (0.04)

[a] GEE analysis with an exchangeable correlation structure.

Table 10.7. Regression coefficients and standard errors (in parentheses) derived from a random coefficient analysis[a] performed on a complete dataset and several incomplete datasets to investigate the (longitudinal) relationship between the dichotomous outcome variable Y and several predictor variables

	X_1	X_2	X_3	X_4	Time
Complete dataset	0.33 (1.63)	0.72 (0.14)	−0.23 (0.36)	0.46 (0.70)	−0.07 (0.10)
Drop-outs					
Ignorable	0.78 (1.80)	0.87 (0.16)	0.07 (0.73)	−0.03 (0.40)	−0.12 (0.10)
Informative	0.36 (1.90)	0.86 (0.17)	0.35 (0.80)	−0.02 (0.42)	−0.16 (0.11)
Intermittent missing data					
Ignorable	0.46 (1.58)	0.81 (0.16)	−0.15 (0.44)	−0.01 (0.68)	−0.19 (0.09)
Informative	0.74 (1.43)	0.83 (0.17)	0.12 (0.42)	0.18 (0.74)	−0.16 (0.08)

[a] Random coefficient analysis with only a random intercept.

For dichotomous outcome variables, however, the situation is totally different. Tables 10.6 and 10.7 show the results of the GEE analysis and random coefficient analysis on incomplete datasets with a dichotomous outcome variable. Both GEE analysis and random coefficient analysis of the incomplete datasets produce results that are (remarkably) different from the results of the analysis of the complete dataset. The differences are observed in both the regression coefficients and the standard errors. In general, there are no systematic differences between the performance of GEE analysis and random coefficient analysis. Furthermore, there are no systematic differences between the results of the analysis of the datasets with ignorable and informative missing data. In fact, the influence of missing data in the analysis of a dichotomous outcome variable is rather unpredictable.

10.5 Comments

Although the examples in the foregoing sections have general implications, it should be noted that in these examples only a few scenarios with missing data were illustrated, while in real life situations infinite patterns of missing data can occur. Furthermore, in the examples only the Y values were presented as missing, while in practice it is just as likely to have missing data in the predictor variables as well. However, based on the results of the examples it can be concluded that GEE analysis and random coefficient analysis behave equally well in the analysis of a dataset with missing data, or equally badly when a dichotomous outcome variable is considered. When the outcome variable was continuous, the results of both GEE analysis and random coefficient analysis performed on a dataset with missing data were comparable to the results obtained from a complete dataset. However, this was not the case for dichotomous outcome variables. Furthermore, there were no major differences between drop-outs and intermittent missing data, and there were no major differences between ignorable and informative missing data. It can also be concluded that performing a MANOVA for repeated measurements on a dataset with missing data is of limited value owing to the removal of all incomplete cases from the analysis.

Because a few decades ago MANOVA for repeated measurements was the only available method for the analysis of longitudinal data, imputation techniques were developed in order to create complete datasets. In the following sections, several of the available imputation methods to replace missing data will be discussed, and the influence of different imputation methods on the results of statistical analysis will be illustrated. This will not be limited to a MANOVA for repeated measurements, but the performance of GEE analysis and random coefficient analysis on imputed datasets will also be evaluated.

10.6 Imputation methods

10.6.1 Continuous outcome variables

Imputation methods can be divided into cross-sectional and longitudinal imputation methods. Both can be used to replace missing data in longitudinal studies. The cross-sectional methods described here are the 'mean or median of series' method, the 'hot-deck' method and the 'cross-sectional linear regression' method. Longitudinal imputation methods which are discussed are the 'last value carried forward' or 'last observation carried forward' method, the 'linear interpolation' method and the 'longitudinal linear regression' method. The 'multiple imputation' method will also be considered.

10.6.1.1 Cross-sectional imputation methods

All variants of the 'mean or median of series' imputation method involve calculation of the average value (mean or median) of the available data for a particular variable at a particular time-point. This average value is imputed for the missing values. Because of its simplicity, it is by far the most frequently used imputation method in practice. A somewhat different approach is called the 'hot-deck' imputation method. With this approach, the average value of (or a random value drawn from) a sub-set of comparable subjects (e.g. subjects with the same gender, age, etc.) is imputed for the missing value. The minimum number of subjects in the sub-set can be one, and the maximum number can be the total population (which makes the 'hot-deck' approach the same as the 'mean/median of series' approach). With 'cross-sectional regression' methods, a linear regression with all available predictor variables at a certain time-point is used to provide predicted values for the outcome variable Y at that particular time-point. This predicted value is used for the imputation. It is obvious that this approach is only suitable in situations when only the outcome variable is missing and not the (possible) predictor variables.

10.6.1.2 Longitudinal imputation methods

The simplest longitudinal imputation method is called the 'last value carried forward' (LVCF) method. In this approach the value of a variable at $t = 1$ for a particular subject is imputed for a missing value for that same subject at $t = 2$. Another longitudinal imputation method is the 'linear interpolation'

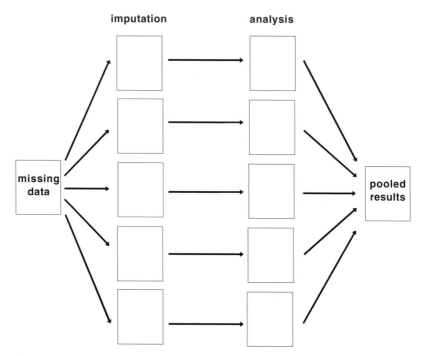

Figure 10.3. Illustration of the multiple imputation technique.

method. With this method, for a missing value at $t = 2$ the average of the values at $t = 1$ and $t = 3$ is imputed, assuming a linear development over time of the variables with missing data. Comparable, but somewhat more sophisticated, is the 'longitudinal regression' imputation method. With this method the linear regression between the outcome variable Y and time is assessed for each subject with a missing value. The predicted value for the time-point of the missing value is imputed for that missing value.

10.6.1.3 Multiple imputation method

With the 'multiple imputation' method, various (say M) imputation values are calculated for every missing value. With the M imputations, M complete datasets are developed, and on each dataset created in this way, statistical analyses are performed. The M complete dataset summary statistics (e.g. regression coefficients) can be combined (i.e. pooled) to form one summary statistic (see Figure 10.3).

The point estimate of the summary statistic is calculated as the average of the M imputations. The variance of the summary statistic is usually calculated from two components. One component reflects the within-imputation variance (the average of the variances of the summary statistics of the M imputations) and the other component reflects the between-imputation variance (the difference between the summary statistic of each imputation and the average of the summary statistics of the M imputations). Equation (10.1) shows a possible way in which the overall variance is calculated:

$$\text{var}_t = \frac{\sum_{i=1}^{M} \text{var}_i}{M} \tag{10.1a}$$

$$\text{var}_b = \frac{\sum_{i=1}^{M} (b_i - \bar{b})^2}{M - 1} \tag{10.1b}$$

$$\text{var} = \text{var}_t + \frac{M + 1}{M} \text{var}_b \tag{10.1c}$$

where var_t is the within-imputation variance, var_i is the variance of imputation i, M is the number of imputations, var_b is the between-imputations variance, b_i is the parameter of interest calculated with imputation i, and $\bar{b}$ is the average of the parameter of interest calculated with M imputations.

The major advantage of the multiple imputation method is that the combined variance is greater than the variance obtained from a single imputation method. This greater variance accounts for the uncertainty introduced by estimating the missing values. In principle, the M imputations of the missing values are M repetitions from the 'posterior predictive distribution' of the missing values. The 'posterior predictive distribution' is related to a 'model for missing data' which can (or in fact must) be based on the information derived from the simple analyses discussed in Sections 10.2 and 10.3. When the missing data are known to be dependent on earlier values of the outcome variable and on the values of several predictor variables, these variables can be used (for instance in a regression analysis) to create the 'posterior predictive distribution' of the missing values (see the example in Section 10.6.3.1). For extensive information on the multiple imputation technique, reference is made to several other publications (e.g. Rubin, 1987, 1996; Schafer, 1997, 1999).

10.6.2 Dichotomous and categorical outcome variables

For dichotomous and/or categorical outcome variables a commonly used cross-sectional method is imputation of the category with the highest frequency for the subject(s) with missing data. This can either be based on the total population ('mean of series' approach) or on a particular sub-set ('hot-deck' approach). The most frequently used longitudinal imputation method available for dichotomous and categorical missing data is the 'LVCF' method. Linear interpolation can be used, but the average value of the outcome variable at the two surrounding time-points has to be rounded off. For dichotomous outcome variables, cross-sectional and longitudinal logistic regression can also be used to predict missing data. However, in these situations the predicted values also have to be rounded off, which makes the use of these techniques slightly complicated.

10.6.3 Example

10.6.3.1 Continuous outcome variables

The influence of missing data and the influence of imputation methods on the results of statistical analysis will be illustrated for MANOVA for repeated measurements and for GEE analysis, and will only be shown for the datasets with intermittent missing data (for an extensive illustration see Twisk and de Vente, 2002).

In this example, one cross-sectional imputation method (i.e. 'mean of series'), one longitudinal imputation method (i.e. 'LVCF') and one multiple imputation technique will be illustrated. For the 'multiple imputation' used in this example, five independent samples from the 'posterior predictive distribution' of the missing values were drawn to form five complete datasets. The 'posterior predictive distribution' was created by an individual linear regression analysis between the outcome variable Y and time. So, for each subject with missing data, a regression analysis with time was performed, based on the observed values for that particular subject. With the estimated regression coefficient and corresponding standard error at each missing data-point, a normal distribution was created with the value estimated by the

Table 10.8. Explained variances and *p*-values (in parentheses) derived from a MANOVA for repeated measurements performed on datasets with imputed missing values

	X_4	Time	Time by X_4
Complete dataset	0.04 ($p = 0.01$)	0.42 ($p < 0.01$)	0.05 ($p < 0.01$)
Ignorable missing data			
Mean	0.04 ($p = 0.02$)	0.37 ($p < 0.01$)	0.03 ($p < 0.01$)
LVCF[a]	0.03 ($p = 0.04$)	0.33 ($p < 0.01$)	0.05 ($p < 0.01$)
Multiple imputation	0.03 ($p = 0.02$)	0.24 ($p < 0.01$)	0.05 ($p < 0.01$)
Informative missing data			
Mean	0.04 ($p = 0.02$)	0.36 ($p < 0.01$)	0.03 ($p < 0.01$)
LVCF[a]	0.03 ($p = 0.03$)	0.37 ($p < 0.01$)	0.05 ($p < 0.01$)
Multiple imputation	0.04 ($p = 0.02$)	0.35 ($p < 0.01$)	0.05 ($p < 0.01$)

[a] LVCF is the last value carried forward.

regression equation as mean value. From this normal distribution, the imputed values are drawn.

Table 10.8 shows the results of the MANOVA for repeated measurements. If the results from Table 10.8 are compared to the results presented in Table 10.3, it can be seen that for the effect of X_4 and the interaction between time and X_4, the results of the imputed datasets are closer to the complete dataset than the results of the incomplete datasets. Furthermore, the different imputation techniques produced comparable results. On the other hand, imputation of missing data led to an under-estimation of the overall time effect (i.e. lower explained variance).

Table 10.9 shows the results of the GEE analysis. Although the overall conclusions (if based on *p*-values) of the GEE analysis for the different predictor variables do not differ between the various datasets, the point estimates and standard errors differ remarkably between the various imputation methods. First of all, it can be seen that the longitudinal imputation method (i.e. LVCF) behaves better than the cross-sectional imputation method (i.e. mean). Furthermore, it can be seen that with the mean imputation technique, the standard errors of the regression coefficients for the time-independent predictors X_1 and X_4 (less pronounced) were under-estimated. This results in smaller confidence intervals and lower

Table 10.9. Regression coefficients and standard errors (in parentheses) derived from a GEE analysis[a] performed on datasets with imputed missing values

	X_1	X_2	X_3	X_4	Time
Complete dataset	−0.02 (0.27)	0.11 (0.02)	−0.11 (0.06)	0.10 (0.11)	0.11 (0.01)
Ignorable missing data					
Mean	0.05 (0.22)	0.11 (0.02)	−0.07 (0.06)	0.05 (0.11)	0.10 (0.01)
LVCF[b]	−0.11 (0.28)	0.10 (0.02)	−0.10 (0.06)	0.05 (0.13)	0.08 (0.01)
Multiple imputation	−0.13 (0.31)	0.10 (0.03)	−0.07 (0.11)	0.04 (0.16)	0.10 (0.03)
Informative missing data					
Mean	0.02 (0.21)	0.10 (0.02)	−0.04 (0.06)	0.05 (0.09)	0.09 (0.01)
LVCF[b]	−0.05 (0.28)	0.09 (0.02)	−0.12 (0.05)	0.09 (0.13)	0.09 (0.01)
Multiple imputation	0.02 (0.33)	0.10 (0.02)	−0.06 (0.07)	0.11 (0.15)	0.10 (0.02)

[a] GEE analysis with an exchangeable correlation structure.
[b] LVCF is the last value carried forward.

p-values, which can lead to incorrect conclusions. This effect was strongest in the dataset with informative missing data. The fact that GEE analysis under-estimates the standard errors of the regression coefficients of the time-independent predictors when cross-sectional imputation methods are applied, has to do with the decreased variance in outcome variable Y, due to the cross-sectional imputation techniques, and with the estimation procedures for time-independent predictor variables in GEE analysis.

The results of the analyses of incomplete datasets (see Table 10.4) were comparable to the results of the analysis of datasets with any of the imputation techniques, so imputation does not seem to be necessary. With the multiple imputation technique, all standard errors were 'over-estimated'. This is caused by the between-imputations variance, which is added as an extra component to the overall variance. The larger standard errors lead to broader confidence intervals and therefore to higher p-values, which is the reason for more conservative conclusions about the relationships analysed. It seems, however, justified that the imputation uncertainty is reflected in the final results of the statistical analyses. The differences in point estimates between multiple imputations and the other imputation methods were not consistent, which can be due to the choice of the (relatively simple) 'model for missing data' used for the multiple imputations, although in general simple (but reasonable) 'models for missing data' are preferable.

Because of its relative simplicity, in the 'applied' literature, the cross-sectional mean is the imputation method most often used. It is important to realize that using the cross-sectional mean imputation method can lead to rather 'strange' results of statistical analysis (see also Twisk and de Vente, 2002).

10.6.3.2 *Dichotomous outcome variables*

In the example with dichotomous outcome variables, three imputation techniques will also be illustrated: one cross-sectional imputation method (i.e. 'category with the highest frequency'), one longitudinal imputation method (i.e. 'LVCF'), and a multiple imputation method. The latter is based on the probability of having a certain value of the outcome variable Y_{dich} for the subject with missing data. So, when a particular subject has one missing value in six measurements, and one at three measurements and zero at the other two measurements, the probability to impute 1 is 0.6 and the probability to impute 0 is 0.4. This procedure is performed for all subjects with missing data and is repeated five times.

Because of the difference between the results of GEE analysis and random coefficient analysis of dichotomous outcome variables (see Chapter 6), both sophisticated techniques will be used to illustrate the 'importance' of imputing missing values. Furthermore, not only the datasets with intermittent missing data but also the datasets with drop-outs will be analysed. A MANOVA for repeated measurements will (of course) not be performed, because this type of analysis can only be carried out for continuous outcome variables (see Chapter 3).

Tables 10.10 and 10.11 show the results of both analyses. When the results of the analysis with imputed datasets are compared to the results obtained from analysis of the datasets with missing values (see Tables 10.6 and 10.7), it must be concluded that the imputation of missing values did not lead to more 'valid' results of the statistical analysis. This is quite surprising, because it was expected that for instance the LVCF method applied to the informative missing datasets would produce results comparable to those obtained from analysis of the complete dataset. For both GEE analysis and random

Table 10.10. Regression coefficients and standard errors (in parentheses) derived from a GEE analysis[a] performed on datasets with imputed missing values with a dichotomous outcome variable

	X_1	X_2	X_3	X_4	Time
Complete dataset	0.22 (0.76)	0.34 (0.06)	−0.15 (0.20)	0.08 (0.37)	−0.08 (0.04)
Ignorable drop-outs					
Highest frequency[b]	0.17 (0.75)	0.38 (0.06)	−0.01 (0.20)	−0.09 (0.37)	−0.17 (0.04)
LVCF[c]	0.10 (0.77)	0.32 (0.06)	−0.03 (0.19)	−0.01 (0.38)	−0.05 (0.04)
Multiple imputation	0.28 (0.78)	0.33 (0.06)	−0.02 (0.20)	0.04 (0.38)	−0.05 (0.04)
Informative drop-outs					
Highest frequency[b]	0.26 (0.66)	0.34 (0.08)	0.07 (0.26)	−0.13 (0.34)	−0.39 (0.06)
LVCF[c]	−0.32 (0.81)	0.26 (0.06)	−0.09 (0.18)	0.15 (0.38)	0.03 (0.04)
Multiple imputation	0.00 (0.80)	0.27 (0.06)	−0.02 (0.18)	0.14 (0.37)	−0.03 (0.04)
Ignorable intermittent missing data					
Highest frequency[b]	0.19 (0.72)	0.40 (0.06)	−0.02 (0.22)	−0.21 (0.36)	−0.09 (0.04)
LVCF[c]	−0.44 (0.79)	0.29 (0.06)	−0.11 (0.17)	−0.04 (0.38)	−0.07 (0.04)
Multiple imputation	0.15 (0.80)	0.30 (0.06)	−0.06 (0.18)	0.11 (0.38)	−0.09 (0.04)
Informative intermittent missing data					
Highest frequency[b]	0.41 (0.58)	0.36 (0.06)	−0.03 (0.21)	−0.03 (0.28)	−0.17 (0.04)
LVCF[c]	0.15 (0.79)	0.34 (0.07)	−0.02 (0.16)	0.05 (0.37)	−0.02 (0.04)
Multiple imputation	0.17 (0.80)	0.29 (0.06)	−0.02 (0.19)	0.13 (0.37)	−0.05 (0.04)

[a] GEE analysis with an exchangeable correlation structure.
[b] Highest frequency is the category with the highest frequency.
[c] LVCF is the last value carried forward.

coefficient analysis this is, however, far from true. Due to the 'robustness' of GEE analysis in a longitudinal analysis with dichotomous outcome variables and the (relative) 'non-robustness' of random coefficient analysis (see Chapter 6 and Chapter 12), it was furthermore expected that the results of the GEE analysis would be 'better' than the results obtained from random coefficient analysis. However, this was also not true in the example presented. Neither did the multiple imputation method lead to 'better' results.

In general, there are distortions in the results of the analyses of both incomplete datasets and the imputed datasets, which makes the interpretation of these results very problematic. In fact, the results of the analyses performed

Table 10.11. Regression coefficients and standard errors (in parentheses) derived from a random coefficient analysis[a] performed on datasets with imputed missing values with a dichotomous outcome variable

	X_1	X_2	X_3	X_4	Time
Complete dataset	0.88 (1.81)	0.70 (0.14)	−0.25 (0.36)	0.34 (0.71)	−0.16 (0.07)
Ignorable drop-outs					
Highest frequency[b]	0.18 (1.73)	0.65 (0.13)	0.02 (0.37)	−0.05 (0.61)	−0.31 (0.08)
LVCF[c]	−0.49 (1.53)	0.79 (0.16)	−0.10 (0.40)	−0.09 (0.77)	−0.13 (0.08)
Multiple imputation	1.02 (2.17)	0.75 (0.16)	−0.01 (0.38)	0.37 (0.91)	−0.13 (0.07)
Informative drop-outs					
Highest frequency[b]	0.34 (0.92)	0.47 (0.10)	0.10 (0.32)	−0.08 (0.40)	−0.51 (0.07)
LVCF[c]	−1.13 (1.86)	0.72 (0.16)	−0.17 (0.46)	−0.30 (0.71)	0.06 (0.08)
Multiple imputation	1.00 (1.92)	0.58 (0.16)	0.01 (0.42)	0.11 (1.09)	−0.04 (0.08)
Ignorable intermittent missing data					
Highest frequency[b]	0.48 (1.12)	0.60 (0.11)	−0.04 (0.32)	−0.12 (0.46)	−0.13 (0.07)
LVCF[c]	0.20 (1.03)	0.70 (0.12)	−0.19 (0.36)	−0.57 (0.51)	−0.15 (0.08)
Multiple imputation	1.48 (2.00)	0.59 (0.13)	−0.19 (0.39)	0.28 (0.60)	−0.08 (0.10)
Informative intermittent missing data					
Highest frequency[b]	0.48 (0.71)	0.42 (0.08)	−0.03 (0.28)	0.00 (0.31)	−0.20 (0.06)
LVCF[c]	0.78 (1.23)	1.00 (0.16)	0.11 (0.37)	−0.36 (0.53)	−0.09 (0.07)
Multiple imputation	1.20 (1.61)	0.58 (0.15)	0.00 (0.44)	−0.23 (0.84)	−0.10 (0.07)

[a] Random coefficient analysis with only a random intercept.
[b] Highest frequency is the category with the highest frequency.
[c] LVCF is the last value carried forward.

on missing datasets and imputed datasets are another illustration of the instability of longitudinal analysis with dichotomous outcome variables.

10.6.4 Comments

It should be noted that in the foregoing examples only a few imputation methods have been illustrated, whereas many more models for imputation are available. The multiple imputation methods were, for instance, limited to (relatively) simple models and (only) five replications of the imputed values. One should be aware of these limitations when evaluating the results of the different imputation methods. Another important issue is that the choice of dataset for the example partly determines the performance of the different imputation techniques. For instance, the stronger the relationship between the predictor variables and the outcome variable Y, the better the imputation methods using these predictor variables will behave. When the outcome variable Y does not change very much over time, the performance of longitudinal imputation methods using the information of Y at earlier time-points will be better. In general, one should be aware of the choices that have been made when evaluating the results of the examples illustrating the different imputation methods.

It has been argued that using imputations for missing data results in a decrease in variability of that particular variable. In theory, this is quite obvious for the mean of series and the hot-deck approach, but a decrease in variability is also a problem in the regression approaches, in which all imputed values lie exactly on the estimated regression line. To overcome this problem, a value can be imputed that is randomly chosen from a range of values, for instance from the normal distribution around the predicted mean value (as in the multiple imputation example for a continuous outcome variable).

In theory, the multiple imputation method is the most elegant solution for the imputation of missing data. However, the performance of the multiple imputation method is highly dependent on the chosen model for missing data. In the example, the results derived from the multiple-imputed dataset showed no difference in regression coefficients compared to the single-imputed datasets. The difference was found in 'better' (i.e. higher) standard errors of the regression coefficients. It is possible that if more sophisticated models for missing data were used, the performance of the 'multiple imputation' method would be better, in such a way that the point estimates would be closer to the point estimates derived from the complete dataset. However, this is highly questionable. With specific software, such as SOLAS (1997), NORM (1999), and the SAS procedure MI (SAS Institute Inc., 2001), more complicated models for missing data can be used for multiple imputation. It is also argued that with the multiple imputation method, the uncertainty of the model for missing data can be added to the estimation. This can be done by taking the imputations of missing data from different models of missing data instead of from only one model (see, for instance, Rubin, 1996).

10.7 Alternative approaches

In Sections 10.5 and 10.6, several imputation methods that can be used to replace missing data have been discussed. Replacing missing data is, however, not the only solution to the problem of missing data. Many alternative approaches are suggested. In the field of epidemiology, it is often suggested that a GEE analysis should be performed, correcting for missing data by adding a dummy variable (missing versus not missing) to the statistical model. This would lead to a less biased estimation of the regression coefficients (e.g. Haan et al., 1999). However, it is questionable whether this approach is very useful. Greenland and Finkle (1995), for instance, caution against indicators for missing data on covariates, and perhaps similar warnings may apply to indicators for missing data on the outcome variable.

A different approach, that is suitable for experimental studies, is suggested by Shih and Quan (1997). They suggest combining the results of two analyses: (1) comparison of the outcome variable between the groups analysed for the subjects with complete data and (2) comparison of the percentage of outcome-related drop-outs between the groups analysed. The p-values of these two analyses can be combined to give the p-value for the 'real' difference between the groups.

In the literature, many other alternative approaches are suggested (e.g. Little, 1993, 1994; Fitzmaurice et al., 1994; Hogan and Laird, 1997; Molenberghs et al., 1998; Kenward, 1998; Kenward and Molenberghs, 1999; Chen et al., 2000; Verbeke and Molenberghs, 2000; Sun and Song, 2001), but unfortunately most of them are very technical and difficult to understand for non-statisticians. Little (1995) provides an extensive overview of modelling drop-out mechanisms, but this review is also rather technical.

10.8 Conclusions

For continuous outcome variables, the use of imputation methods is recommended when MANOVA for repeated measurements is used to analyse a longitudinal dataset with missing data. When more sophisticated methods (i.e. GEE analysis or random coefficient analysis) are used to analyse a longitudinal dataset with missing data, no imputations at all may be better than applying any of the imputation methods. If a decision is made to impute missing values, longitudinal methods are generally preferred above cross-sectional methods. In the example dataset presented in this chapter, the more refined multiple imputation method of imputing missing values did not lead to any difference in the point estimates, compared to the single imputation techniques. The estimated standard errors were higher in the datasets with missing values than in the complete dataset, which certainly seems to reflect uncertainty in estimation caused by imputing missing values.

For dichotomous outcome variables, it is recommended that there should be no missing values! The results of the analysis of both incomplete datasets and datasets with imputed values are (highly) unpredictable, and should be interpreted with the utmost caution.

11

Tracking

11.1 Introduction

In the epidemiological literature, tracking is used to describe the relative stability of the longitudinal development of a certain outcome variable Y. There is no single widely accepted definition of tracking, but the following concepts are involved: (1) the relationship (correlation) between early measurements and measurements later in life, or the maintenance of a relative position within a distribution of values in the observed population over time, and (2) the predictability of future values by early measurements (Ware and Wu, 1981; Twisk et al., 1994). In epidemiology, tracking is mainly used in the assessment of risk factors for chronic diseases (Clarke et al., 1978; Lauer et al., 1986; Hibbert et al., 1990; Porkka et al., 1991: Lee et al., 1992; Beunen et al., 1992; Casey et al., 1992; Twisk et al., 1997, 1998a, 1998b, 2000). The early detection of risk factors can lead to the possibility of early treatment. In this respect, it is important to estimate the stability of a certain risk factor over time: 'What is the relationship between measurements of risk factors early in life and values of the same risk factors at a later date?', 'How predictive are early measurements for values later in life?' There are many different ways to analyse tracking, and in this chapter a summary will be given of the (basic) methods of assessment.

11.2 Continuous outcome variables

When there are only two measurements, the simplest way to assess tracking or stability is to calculate a Pearson correlation coefficient. The Pearson correlation coefficient is only suitable when both Y at $t = 1$ and Y at $t = 2$ are normally distributed. When the data are not normally distributed, Spearman's rank correlation coefficient (i.e. the Pearson correlation coefficient calculated for rank numbers of the original variables) can be used for tracking.

When there are more than two longitudinal measurements, the problem with using a simple Pearson correlation coefficient for tracking is that it does not use all the available data, or that several correlation coefficients are needed to describe tracking over the entire longitudinal period. When Y at $t = 1$ to Y at $t = T$ are all normally distributed with equal variances and covariances, a possible solution to this problem is to calculate the intraclass correlation coefficient (ICC), which is (usually) defined as:

$$\text{ICC} = \frac{\left(\sigma_B^2 - \sigma_W^2\right)}{\left(\sigma_B^2 + \sigma_W^2\right)} \tag{11.1}$$

where σ_B^2 is the between-subjects variance, and σ_W^2 is the within-subject variance.

When Y at $t = 1$ to Y at $t = T$ are not normally distributed, Kendall's coefficient of concordance (W) can be calculated. This coefficient is a measure of stability based on rank numbers of the outcome variable (i.e. on changes in individual rankings over time).

$$W = \frac{12}{T^2 \, N(N+1)(N-1)} \sum_{i=1}^{N} \left[R_i - \frac{T(N+1)}{2} \right]^2 \tag{11.2}$$

where T is the number of measurements, N is the number of subjects, and R_i is the sum of all rankings at all measurements for individual i.

Kendall's W can take values between 0.0 and 1.0, and indicates the degree of association between the rankings at each of the repeated measurements. However, the interpretation of W is quite complicated, because when W is calculated for random numbers the coefficient is not equal to zero, but to a positive value which depends on the number of time-points T.

Foulkes and Davis (1981) have developed a tracking coefficient γ for longitudinal studies when $T \geq 2$. In their approach, the observed values for each subject are replaced by the predicted values obtained from individual regression analyses between the outcome variable Y and time. These regression functions can be either linear (straight lines) or more complicated, and can be seen as individual growth lines or curves. The Foulkes and Davis tracking coefficient γ, also known as the growth separation index, is used to determine the probability that two subjects selected at random will have growth lines or curves that do not cross during the time period under consideration. This probability is simply the number of growth lines or curves in the population that do not cross, divided by the number of ways in which two lines or curves can be randomly selected from the population:

$$\gamma[t_1, t_T] = 1 - \sum_{i=1}^{N} \frac{m_i}{N(N-1)} \tag{11.3}$$

where m_i is the number of times the growth line or curve of a particular subject crosses at least once with the growth lines or curves of other subjects during the observed time period $[t_1, t_T]$, and N is the number of subjects.

As for all other tracking indices, the value of γ highly depends on the length of the observed time period. The coefficient γ can take values between 0.0 and 1.0. A value of 0.0 means that every individual line or curve crosses every other individual line or curve at least once; a value of 1.0 indicates that none of the individual lines or curves cross; a value >0.5 indicates tracking, because two subjects chosen at random would be more likely to have lines or curves that do not cross. When the individual response patterns are simply drawn by connecting the successive time-points, without assuming any mathematical growth model, this procedure would be based on rank numbers. Although there are no assumptions about the form of the lines or curves, the simplicity of the model used to describe the data is very important. In other words: the simpler the model used to describe the data, the higher is the value of the tracking coefficient. Another problem in interpreting γ is that subjects at the extremes of the distribution are less likely to have lines that cross the lines or curves of other subjects than subjects who have lines or curves near the mean line or curve. If measurements are made at only two points in time, and therefore the lines or curves for each subject are straight lines, then the Foulkes and Davis tracking coefficient γ is equivalent to Spearman's rank correlation coefficient.

McMahan (1981) has developed a tracking coefficient τ, which is also based on all the available data. The coefficient is calculated under the assumption that all repeated measurements of outcome variable Y are normally distributed. The McMahan tracking coefficient, which is also known as the growth constancy index, is calculated as follows:

$$\tau = 1 - \frac{1}{(N-1)(T-1)} \sum_{i=1}^{N} S_i^2 \qquad (11.4a)$$

$$S_i^2 = \sum_{t=1}^{T} (Y_{it} - \bar{Y}_i)^2 \qquad (11.4b)$$

$$\bar{Y}_i = \frac{1}{T} \sum_{t=1}^{T} Y_{it} \qquad (11.4c)$$

where N is the number of subjects, T is the number of repeated measurements, and Y_{it} is the observation for individual i at time-point t.

Basically, τ is nothing more than the average value of the $(T(T-1))/2$ Pearson correlation coefficients, where T is the number of times a value is measured. If τ has a value of 1.0, there is perfect tracking for that variable. If τ has a value of 0.0, there is no tracking for that variable. Like the Pearson correlation coefficient, McMahan's τ can take negative values, which indicates a reversal of the values between two observed time-points.

Another possibility is to use longitudinal principal component (LPC) analysis to assess tracking in a certain continuous outcome variable Y over time. Assuming a linear relationship between the repeated measurements, LPC analysis starts by finding the linear combination of the same variable measured on different occasions, which accounts for the maximum amount of variance. This linear combination is called the first principal component. The percentage of variance (R^2) accounted for by the first principal component can be interpreted as a tracking coefficient.

One of the latest innovations in the assessment of tracking is a more general method in which the tracking coefficient is calculated with the following statistical model:

$$Y_{it} = \beta_0 + \beta_1 Y_{it1} + \beta_2 t + \sum_{j=1}^{J} \beta_{3j} X_{ijt} + \sum_{k=1}^{K} \beta_{4k} Z_{ik} + \varepsilon_{it} \qquad (11.5)$$

where Y_{it} are observations for subject i at time t, β_0 is the intercept, Y_{it1} is the initial (first) observation for subject i, β_1 is the regression coefficient used as tracking coefficient, t is time, β_2 is the regression coefficient for time, X_{ijt} is the time-dependent covariate j of individual i, β_{3j} is the regression coefficient for time-dependent covariate j, J is the number of time-dependent covariates, Z_{ik} is the time-independent covariate k for subject i, β_{4k} is the regression coefficient for time-independent covariate k, K is the number of time-independent covariates, and ε_{it} is the 'error' for subject i at time-point t.

To calculate a tracking coefficient for a certain outcome variable Y, the value of the initial measurement at $t_1 (Y_{it1})$ is regressed on the entire longitudinal development of that variable from t_2 to t_T. The relationships between the initial value at t_1 and the values from t_2 to t_T are analysed simultaneously, resulting in one single regression coefficient (β_1). The standardized value of this coefficient can be interpreted as a longitudinal correlation coefficient, i.e. the tracking coefficient.

The regression coefficient (β_1) can easily be standardized by applying Equation (11.6):

$$\beta_s = \frac{\beta \operatorname{sd}(X)}{\operatorname{sd}(Y)} \tag{11.6}$$

where β_s is the standardized regression coefficient, β is the non-standardized regression coefficient, $\operatorname{sd}(X)$ is the standard deviation of the predictor variable, and $\operatorname{sd}(Y)$ is the standard deviation of the outcome variable.

Although this tracking coefficient can range between -1 and $+1$, assuming the correlations between the repeated observations to be positive, this tracking coefficient takes values between 0 and 1. The statistical model is comparable to the model described to analyse the longitudinal relationship between a continuous outcome variable and one or more predictor variables (see Section 4.4, Equation (4.3)). The only difference is that the initial value of the outcome variable (Y_{it1}) is one of the predictor variables. The regression coefficient of interest (β_1) can be estimated in exactly the same way as has been described before, i.e. by means of GEE analysis or random coefficient analysis. The way the tracking coefficient is estimated according to Equation (11.5) is illustrated below:

$$\begin{bmatrix} Y_2 \\ Y_3 \\ Y_4 \\ Y_5 \\ Y_6 \end{bmatrix} = \beta_0 + \beta_1 \begin{bmatrix} Y_1 \\ Y_1 \\ Y_1 \\ Y_1 \\ Y_1 \end{bmatrix} + \beta_2 \begin{bmatrix} X_2 \\ X_3 \\ X_4 \\ X_5 \\ X_6 \end{bmatrix} \cdots$$

One of the greatest advantages of this model is the fact that all longitudinal data are used to calculate one tracking coefficient. Furthermore, this method is suitable for highly unbalanced longitudinal datasets, i.e. a different number of repeated measurements for each subject and unequally spaced time intervals. A third advantage is the possibility to correct for both time-dependent (X_{itj}) and time-independent covariates (Z_{ik}). These covariates can be continuous, as well as dichotomous or categorical. A comparable approach is the use of an autoregressive model (see Section 5.2.3, Equation (5.3)). The autoregression coefficient can be interpreted as a tracking coefficient. However, the interpretation is somewhat different from the tracking coefficient estimated with Equation (11.5), because the autoregression coefficient describes the relationship between the value of a certain outcome variable Y at time-point t and the value of outcome variable Y at $t - 1$, while the β_1 coefficient in the tracking model describes the relationship between the value of Y at t_1 and the total development of Y from t_2 to t_T. The same autoregression coefficient can be estimated with the use of structural equation models (LISREL). The LISREL approach is particularly suitable in situations when a so-called latent (unobserved) variable is analysed (Jöreskog and Sörbom, 1993, 2001). However, these models are sometimes difficult to fit, and the estimations of the coefficients are rather unstable in smaller populations.

11.3 Dichotomous and categorical outcome variables

The simplest way to calculate tracking for dichotomous and categorical outcome variables is to calculate the proportion of subjects in a specific group who stayed in the same group at one or more follow-up measurement(s). If that proportion is higher than the expected proportion when the subjects are randomly divided into each group (e.g. more than 50% for dichotomous variables, more than 25% for four groups, more than 20% for five groups, etc.), the population is said to track for that particular variable.

The same procedure can be carried out for continuous outcome variables, which are divided into percentile groups or into groups according to predetermined cut-off points. By this division, the continuous outcome variable is changed into a dichotomous or categorical outcome variable. Based on these proportions, two corresponding coefficients can be calculated, both of

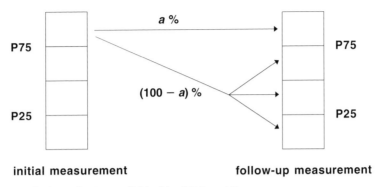

Figure 11.1. 'Predictive value': *a*% divided by (100 − *a*)%.

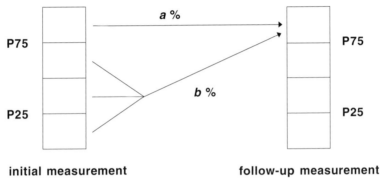

Figure 11.2. 'Relative probability': *a*% divided by *b*%.

which are only suitable in research situations where $T = 2$. The 'predictive value' is calculated as the proportion of subjects who stayed in a certain group during follow-up, divided by the proportion of subjects who moved to other groups (Figure 11.1), and the 'relative probability' is calculated as the proportion of subjects who were in a certain group at the initial measurement as well as at the follow-up measurement, divided by the proportion of subjects who moved from one of the other groups at the initial measurement to that group at the follow-up measurement (Figure 11.2). The term 'relative probability' is somewhat misleading; it is not really a probability, because the value can be greater than one.

Another interesting, possible way to assess tracking for dichotomous and categorical outcome variables is Cohen's kappa (κ), which can be calculated in longitudinal studies where $T \geq 2$. Kappa is calculated as shown in Equation (11.7):

$$\kappa = \frac{\bar{p} - \hat{p}}{1 - \hat{p}} \tag{11.7a}$$

$$\bar{p} = \frac{1}{N} \sum_{i=1}^{N} p_i \tag{11.7b}$$

$$p_i = \frac{1}{T(T-1)} \sum_{g=1}^{G} n_{ig}(n_{ig} - 1) \tag{11.7c}$$

$$\hat{p} = \sum_{g=1}^{G} p_g^2 \tag{11.7d}$$

$$p_g = \frac{1}{NT} \sum_{i=1}^{N} n_{ig} \tag{11.7e}$$

where $\bar{p}$ is the expected proportion of stability, N is the number of subjects, $\hat{p}$ is the observed proportion of stability, G is the number of groups (i.e. two in the case of a dichotomous outcome variable), T is the number of measurements, and n_{ig} is the number of times subject i is in the g group.

The number of times that each individual subject is in each specific group is counted and compared with the value that is expected if the subjects are randomly assigned to the different groups at each measurement. Generally, kappa ranges from 0.0 to 1.0, and if kappa > 0.75, it is considered that the variable tracks well. If kappa < 0.40, then the variable is considered to track poorly, and if the kappa value lies between these two, then there is moderate tracking for the variable of interest. However, these thresholds are rather arbitrary, and as in the case of all other tracking coefficients, the magnitude of kappa is highly influenced by the length of the measurement period. When kappa is calculated for categorical variables, one of the problems is that all 'movements' between groups are weighted equally, irrespective of the length of the 'movement'. To overcome this drawback, Cohen (1968) also developed a weighted kappa, in which the lengths of the movements are weighted unequally (Equation (11.8)). Unfortunately, the weighted index can only be used in situations when there are only two measurements.

$$\kappa = \frac{\bar{p}_w - \hat{p}_w}{1 - \hat{p}_w} \tag{11.8a}$$

$$\bar{p}_w = \sum_{i=1}^{G} \sum_{j=1}^{G} w_{ij} p_{ij} \tag{11.8b}$$

$$\hat{p}_w = \sum_{i=1}^{G} \sum_{j=1}^{G} w_{ij} p_{i(t1)} p_{j(t2)} \tag{11.8c}$$

$$w_{ij} = 1 - \frac{|i - j|}{G - 1} \tag{11.8d}$$

where $\bar{p}_w$ is the (weighted) expected proportion of stability, $\hat{p}_w$ is the (weighted) observed proportion of stability, p_{ii} is the proportion of subjects in a certain group at $t = 1$ and in the same group at $t = 2$, and G is the number of groups (i.e. categories).

Comparable to the method that has been described for continuous outcome variables, a longitudinal logistic regression analysis can also be used to assess tracking for a dichotomous outcome variable, for which the following statistical model can be used:

$$\ln\left[\frac{\Pr(Y_{it} = 1)}{1 - \Pr(Y_{it} = 1)}\right] = \beta_0 + \beta_1 Y_{it1} + \beta_2 t + \sum_{j=1}^{J} \beta_{3j} X_{itj} + \sum_{k=1}^{K} \beta_{4k} Z_{ik} \tag{11.9a}$$

or in another notation

$$\Pr(Y_{it} = 1) = \frac{1}{1 + \exp\left[-\left(\beta_0 + \beta_1 Y_{it1} + \beta_2 t + \sum_{j=1}^{J} \beta_{3j} X_{itj} + \sum_{k=1}^{K} \beta_{4k} Z_{ik}\right)\right]} \tag{11.9b}$$

where $\Pr(Y_{it} = 1)$ is the probability that the observations at t_2 to t_T of subject i equal 1 (where T is the number of measurements and 1 means that subject i belongs to the group of interest), Y_{it1} is the initial (first) observation of subject i at t_1, β_0 is the intercept, β_1 is the regression coefficient used as tracking coefficient, t is time, β_2 is the regression coefficient for time, X_{itj} is the time-dependent covariate j for subject i, β_{3j} is the regression coefficient for time-dependent covariate j, J is the number of time-dependent covariates, Z_{ik} is the time-independent covariate k for subject i, β_{4k} is the regression coefficient for time-dependent covariate k, and K is the number of time-independent covariates.

This model is more or less the same as the model described to analyse the relationship between a dichotomous outcome variable and one or more predictor variables (see Chapter 6, Equations (6.6a) and (6.6b)). The difference is that in the tracking model the probability of belonging to a group from t_2 to t_T is related to the initial membership of the group at t_1 (Y_{it1}). Furthermore, the model has the same advantages as have been described for the model used to calculate the tracking coefficients for continuous outcome variables (Equation (11.5)). The coefficient of interest is β_1, because this coefficient reflects the relationship between belonging to a group at t_1 and the development of that particular group from t_2 to t_T, which is in fact the definition of tracking. Like in simple logistic regression, this coefficient (β_1) can be transformed into an odds ratio ($\exp(\beta_1)$), which gives the magnitude of the 'odds' of a subject belonging to a group at t_1, regarding the development of the subject's group status from t_2 to t_T, relative to the 'odds' of a subject not belonging to that group at t_1. As for continuous outcome variables, the regression coefficients of the tracking model can be estimated with GEE analysis as well as with random coefficient analysis, although GEE analysis is preferred because it provides a so-called 'population-averaged' estimation of the regression coefficients.

For the estimation of tracking for categorical outcome variables, longitudinal polytomous logistic regression analysis can be used, while for the estimation of tracking for a 'count' outcome variable, longitudinal Poisson regression can be used (see Sections 7.1.5.3 and 7.2). Both analyses can use the same extension as was described for continuous and dichotomous outcome variables, i.e. with the initial value of the categorical or 'count' outcome variable at $t = 1$ as one of the predictor variables.

11.4 Example

In the examples, a distinction will be made between research situations with only two measurements and situations with more than two measurements. In the first example, the first and the last measurements of the example dataset

Table 11.1. Tracking coefficients[a] calculated for a continuous outcome variable Y measured twice in time (at $t = 1$ and $t = 6$)

Pearson's correlation coefficient	0.59
Spearman's correlation coefficient	0.63
Intraclass correlation coefficient[b]	0.32 (0.17–0.46)
Kendall's W	0.37
McMahan's tracking coefficient	0.59
Principal component analysis	0.79
Stability coefficient[b]	0.59 (0.45–0.72)

[a] The Foulkes and Davies tracking coefficient cannot be calculated with any of the major commercial software packages, so this coefficient is left out of the example.
[b] The 95% confidence interval is given in parentheses.

will be considered, while in the latter example, all six measurements of the example dataset will be considered.

11.4.1 Two measurements

Table 11.1 shows the results of the different tracking coefficients calculated for the continuous outcome variable Y. Although all coefficients reported in Table 11.1 are intended to measure the same construct and are applied to the same dataset, it is obvious that the magnitude of the tracking coefficient highly depends on the method used.

For a dichotomous outcome variable with only two measurements, all tracking coefficients can be calculated from the following 2×2 table:

		t_6		
		1	2	Total
t_1	1	80	17	97
	2	18	32	50
	Total	98	49	147

Table 11.2 shows the tracking coefficients calculated for a dichotomous outcome variable. From the results it can be seen that (comparable to the situation for continuous outcome variables) the magnitude of the tracking coefficient highly depends on the method used.

Table 11.2. Tracking coefficients calculated for a dichotomous outcome variable Y measured twice in time (at $t = 1$ and $t = 6$)

Proportion of stability	76%
Predictive value[b]	1.78
Relative probability[b]	3.66
Kappa	0.47
Stability coefficient (odds ratio)[a]	8.37 (3.83–18.24)

[a] The 95% confidence interval is given in parentheses.
[b] Based on the second group.

Table 11.3. Tracking coefficients calculated for a categorical outcome variable Y measured twice in time (at $t = 1$ and $t = 6$)

Proportion of stability	55%
Predictive value[b]	1.78
Relative probability[b]	3.66
Kappa	0.33
Weighted kappa[a]	0.34

[a] Weighted kappa is not given in most standard software packages.
[b] Based on the second group.

For a categorical variable with two repeated measurements over time, the tracking coefficients can be calculated directly from the following 3×3 table:

		t_6			
		1	2	3	Total
t_1	1	30	15	3	48
	2	16	19	14	49
	3	3	15	32	50
	Total	49	49	49	147

Table 11.3 shows the tracking coefficients for the categorical outcome variable Y, measured at $t = 1$ and at $t = 6$. When the results from Tables 11.2 and 11.3 are compared, it can be seen that the magnitude of the tracking coefficient depends not only on the method used, but also on the way the outcome variable is categorized (see Section 11.5.3).

Table 11.4. Tracking coefficients[a] calculated for a continuous outcome variable Y measured six times using all available data

Intraclass correlation coefficient[b]	0.54 (0.47–0.62)
Kendall's W	0.34
McMahan's tracking coefficient	0.70
Principal component analysis	0.75
Stability coefficient[b, c]	0.60 (0.53–0.67)

[a] The Foulkes and Davies tracking coefficient cannot be calculated with any of the major commercial software packages, so this coefficient is left out of the example.
[b] The 95% confidence interval is given in parentheses.
[c] Estimated with GEE analysis.

Table 11.5. Tracking coefficients calculated for a dichotomous outcome variable Y measured six times using all available data

Kappa[a]	0.51
Stability coefficient (odds ratio)[b]	8.92 (5.13–15.51)

[a] In a situation with more than two measurements, kappa has to be calculated manually.
[b] Estimated with GEE analysis; the 95% confidence interval is given in parentheses.

11.4.2 More than two measurements

In the following examples, all six measurements are used to estimate the tracking coefficients. Table 11.4 shows the results of the different tracking coefficients calculated for the continuous outcome variable Y. When the tracking coefficients are estimated using all available longitudinal data, most coefficients are similar to those estimated using only the first and last measurements (see Table 11.1). Some of the coefficients are slightly higher when all longitudinal data are used, which is expected because information regarding shorter time periods is used in the estimation. Furthermore, the precision of the estimates is greater in the situation when all available data are used, which is expressed in the smaller confidence intervals of the tracking coefficients.

Table 11.5 shows the tracking coefficients calculated for a dichotomous outcome variable, and Table 11.6 shows the tracking coefficient calculated for a categorical outcome variable. In both situations, all available data (i.e. six measurements) are used to estimate the coefficients. For these kinds of

Table 11.6. Tracking coefficient calculated for a categorical outcome variable Y measured six times using all available data

Kappa[a]	0.41

[a] In a situation with more than two measurements, kappa has to be calculated manually.

outcome variables, the comparison between tracking coefficients estimated with all available data and tracking coefficients estimated with only two measurements is the same as has been described for continuous outcome variables. Furthermore, the magnitude of the tracking coefficients (i.e. kappa) depends on the cut-off value of the categorization, a phenomenon which was already observed in the situation when tracking coefficients were calculated using only two measurements over time.

11.5 Comments

11.5.1 Interpretation of tracking coefficients

One of the major problems in tracking analysis is the interpretation of the results. Conclusions about the tracking phenomenon are mainly based on the significance of the tracking coefficient. The importance of a significance test for the tracking coefficient is, however, very doubtful. This is primarily due to the fact that the statistical significance of the tracking coefficient is based on the hypothesis that the tracking coefficient equals zero. When a tracking coefficient differs significantly from zero, this does not imply that the tracking coefficient for that particular variable is good. Significantly different from zero does not provide any information about the magnitude of the coefficient. Secondly, it is important to realize that the magnitude of every tracking coefficient highly depends on the length of the time interval. A high tracking coefficient calculated over a short time period is not necessarily 'better' than a lower tracking coefficient calculated over a much longer time period. The same problem in interpretation arises when authors wish to evaluate their tracking coefficient by stating that if their tracking coefficient is above a certain value the population tracks for that variable. For instance, kappa > 0.75 indicates tracking, but if the index is calculated over a very short time period, it does not indicate anything. In evaluating tracking coefficients, the magnitude of the point estimate, the width of the 95% confidence interval of the coefficient (which gives information about the precision of the estimate) and the time period over which the coefficient is calculated have to be considered.

Moreover, one must take into account the fact that tracking coefficients are highly influenced by measurement error. If the assessment of a certain outcome variable Y is not very accurate, i.e. if the reproducibility of the measurement of variable Y is rather low, this will probably lead to low tracking coefficients. Low reproducibility of the measurement instrument should be taken into account when interpreting the magnitude of the tracking coefficients.

11.5.2 Risk factors for chronic diseases

One of the major issues that tracking analysis is used to evaluate is the longitudinal development of risk factors for chronic diseases. Before interpreting the tracking coefficient or predictive value, one has to be aware of the fact that the maintenance of a relatively high value of a risk factor over time may not be as important in predicting the development of a disease as a certain increase in this value. That is probably the reason why sometimes not only the proportion of subjects who maintained a certain rank order is calculated, but also the proportion of subjects with a rising rank order (see for instance Lauer et al., 1986). Somewhat related is the fact that tracking concerns the relative position of a certain individual within a group of subjects over time. When tracking is high for a certain variable over time, this does not necessarily mean that the absolute level of that variable does not change over time. When for each individual in a particular population the value of a certain variable Y increases with the same amount, the stability of that variable is very high. In other words, the interpretation of the tracking coefficient is rather relative.

11.5.3 Grouping of continuous outcome variables

If a continuous outcome variable Y is arbitrarily divided into sub-groups (e.g. tertiles or quartiles), the magnitude of the tracking coefficient highly depends on the (arbitrary) decision about how the population is divided (see Section 11.4). This makes these approaches very troublesome in assessing the tracking phenomenon. Furthermore, by dividing the population into sub-groups, a lot of information about the data is lost. For instance, subjects can change position within their original (percentile) group without influencing the tracking coefficient, whereas a minor shift at the borders between two (percentile) groups will influence tracking coefficients.

11.6 Conclusions

It is not the intention of this chapter to recommend a 'perfect' tracking coefficient or a 'perfect' model to assess tracking. The main purpose of this chapter is merely to draw attention to some important aspects of tracking analysis.

On the one hand it is preferable to use a tracking coefficient that is as simple as possible. However, on the other hand, tracking is part of the description of the longitudinal development of a certain variable and, therefore, the approach must include the possibility of using all the available longitudinal data and, if necessary, of controlling for possible confounding variables. Finally it should be kept in mind that the tracking coefficient must be easy to interpret, and that it is very dangerous to give strict rules for the interpretation of tracking coefficients, in particular because the value of a coefficient depends highly on the time period under consideration.

Software for longitudinal data analysis

12.1 Introduction

In the foregoing chapters many research questions have been addressed and many techniques for the analysis of longitudinal data have been discussed. In the examples, the 'simple' statistical techniques were performed with SPSS, while the GEE analyses were performed with SPIDA, and the random coefficient analyses with STATA. Until recently, with the widely used software package SPSS there were not many possibilities of performing sophisticated longitudinal data analysis. However, with the release of SPSS version 11, random coefficient analysis for continuous outcome variables became available. This chapter provides an overview of a few major software packages (i.e. STATA, SAS, S-PLUS, SPSS and MLwiN) and their ability to perform sophisticated longitudinal data analysis. In this chapter, only GEE analysis and random coefficient analysis will be discussed. MANOVA for repeated measurements can be performed with all major software packages, and can usually be found under the repeated measurements option of the generalized linear model (GLM) or as an extension of the (M)ANOVA procedure. The emphasis of this overview lies on the output and syntax of the sophisticated longitudinal analysis in the different software packages, and especially on comparison of the results obtained with the various different packages. In this overview, only analysis with a continuous and a dichotomous outcome variable will be discussed in detail.

12.2 GEE analysis with continuous outcome variables

12.2.1 STATA

Output 12.1 shows the results of a linear GEE analysis (i.e. with a continuous outcome variable) performed with STATA. The first part of the output

Output 12.1. Results of a linear GEE analysis performed with STATA

```
GEE population-averaged model           Number of obs      =       882
Group variable:                    id   Number of groups   =       147
Link:                        identity   Obs per group: min =         6
Family:                      Gaussian                  avg =       6.0
Correlation:             exchangeable                  max =         6
                                        Wald chi2(5)       =    208.03
Scale parameter:            0.5586134   Prob > chi2        =    0.0000
-----------------------------------------------------------------------
ycont       Coeff  Std. Err.      z    P > |z|    [95% Conf. Interval]
-----------------------------------------------------------------------
   x1   -0.0237166   0.276071   -0.086   0.932   -0.5648058   0.5173727
   x2    0.1109326  0.0201324    5.510   0.000    0.0714738   0.1503914
   x3   -0.1108512  0.0584746   -1.896   0.058   -0.2254592   0.0037569
   x4    0.1008476  0.1216047    0.829   0.407   -0.1374932   0.3391885
 time    0.1084771  0.0111322    9.744   0.000    0.0866583   0.1302958
_cons    3.616689   0.6729413    5.374   0.000    2.297748    4.93563
```

provides general information regarding the analysis performed. It can be seen that an identity link is used, which indicates that a linear GEE analysis has been performed. The latter can also be seen from 'Family: Gaussian'. Furthermore, the output shows that an exchangeable correlation structure was used, and that the scale parameter is 0.5586134. On the right-hand side of the general information a Wald statistic and the corresponding p-value are shown (Wald chi2(5) and prob > chi2). This refers to the generalized Wald statistic, which shows the significance of the combination of the five predictor variables in the model (i.e. X_1 to X_4 and time). The second part of the output shows the regression coefficients, the standard errors, the z-value (i.e. the regression coefficient divided by its standard error), the corresponding p-value and the 95% confidence interval of the regression coefficient.

The syntax needed to obtain Output 12.1 is very simple:

```
xtgee ycont x1 x2 x3 x4 time, i(id) corr(exch)
```

First the STATA procedure is specified (i.e. **xtgee**), directly followed by the outcome variable and the predictor variables. After the comma, additional information is supplied, i.e. the subject identifier (id) and the 'working' correlation structure (exch).

It should be noted that in STATA the default procedure for the estimation of the standard errors is so-called 'model based'. This is rather strange, because it is generally accepted that the 'robust' estimation procedure of the standard errors is preferred[1] (Liang and Zeger, 1986). To obtain 'robust' standard errors the following syntax can be used:

```
xtgee ycont x1 x2 x3 x4 time, i(id) corr(exch) robust
```

The major difference between the 'model-based' and the 'robust' estimation procedure occurs when an independent correlation structure is used. In fact, with a 'model-based' estimation procedure, the results obtained from the GEE analysis with an independent correlation structure are exactly the same as the results obtained from a naive linear regression analysis in which the dependency of the observations is ignored.

12.2.2 SAS

Within SAS, the GENMOD procedure can be used to perform a GEE analysis. The output of the GENMOD procedure is rather long, and includes for instance the initial parameter estimates. Output 12.2 shows a section of the output of a linear GEE analysis performed with the GENMOD procedure.

From the output it can be seen that a linear GEE analysis has been performed (i.e. a normal distribution, and an identity link function). Furthermore, it can be seen that an exchangeable correlation structure is used. At the end of the output, the parameter estimates are given, i.e. the regression coefficient, the standard error, the 95% confidence interval of the regression coefficient, the z-value (again obtained from the regression coefficient divided by its standard error) and the corresponding p-value.

The syntax needed to perform a GEE analysis with the GENMOD procedure is slightly more complicated than the syntax for STATA:

```
proc genmod data=long.x;
class id;
model ycont = x1 x2 x3 x4 time;
repeated subject=id/type=exch;
run;
```

Each SAS procedure starts with the procedure specification (**proc genmod**) and ends with a **run** statement. The class statement in SAS is needed to

---

[1] 'Robust' estimation of the standard errors is also known as 'Huber' or 'sandwich' estimation.

Output 12.2. Results of a linear GEE analysis performed with the GENMOD procedure in SAS

<pre>
                        The GENMOD Procedure

                        Model Information

    Data Set   LONGBOOK._FIRST_
    Distribution   Normal
    Link Function   Identity
    Dependent Variable   YCONT   OUTCOME VARIABLE Y
    Observations Used   882

                     GEE Model Information

         Correlation Structure   Exchangeable
         Subject Effect   ID (147 levels)
         Number of Clusters   147
         Correlation Matrix Dimension   6
         Maximum Cluster Size   6
         Minimum Cluster Size   6

 Algorithm converged

               Analysis Of GEE Parameter Estimates
               Empirical Standard Error Estimates

                         Standard   95% Confidence
    Parameter   Estimate   Error   Limits   Z   Pr > |Z|
    Intercept   3.6348   0.6793   2.3035   4.9662   5.35   <0.0001
    TIME   0.1076   0.0139   0.0804   0.1348   7.76   <0.0001
    X1   -0.0302   0.2737   -0.5666   0.5063 -0.11   0.9123
    X2   0.1107   0.0228   0.0660   0.1554   4.85   <0.0001
    X3   -0.1135   0.0607   -0.2324   0.0055 -1.87   0.0616
    X4   0.0991   0.1305   -0.1566   0.3548   0.76   0.4475
</pre>

---

indicate that the subject identifier is a categorical variable (class id). In the third line of the syntax the model to be analysed is specified (model ycont = x1 x2 x3 x4 time), and in the fourth line the fact that the subjects are repeatedly measured (repeated subject=id), and that the correlation structure is exchangeable (type=exch).

12.2.3 S-PLUS

GEE analysis cannot be performed in the regular S-PLUS software package. However, a GEE procedure is available which can be implemented in the

Output 12.3. Results of a linear GEE analysis performed with S-PLUS

```
Model:
 Link:                       Identity
 Variance to Mean Relation: Gaussian
 Correlation Structure:      Exchangeable

Coefficients:
             Estimate   Naive S.E.     Naive z   Robust S.E.     Robust z
(Intercept)  3.63483468  0.67241365   5.4056528   0.67926759    5.3511087
        X1  -0.03015058  0.27585764  -0.1092976   0.27371605   -0.1101528
        X2   0.11070982  0.02007973   5.5135106   0.02282241    4.8509267
        X3  -0.11345790  0.05830270  -1.9460145   0.06071048   -1.8688353
        X4   0.09909445  0.12148692   0.8156800   0.13045478    0.7596077
      TIME   0.10759108  0.01109887   9.6938770   0.01386447    7.7601995

Estimated Scale Parameter: 0.5565875
Number of Iterations: 4

Working Correlation
             [,1]        [,2]        [,3]        [,4]        [,5]        [,6]
[1,]    1.0000000   0.5630412   0.5630412   0.5630412   0.5630412   0.5630412
[2,]    0.5630412   1.0000000   0.5630412   0.5630412   0.5630412   0.5630412
[3,]    0.5630412   0.5630412   1.0000000   0.5630412   0.5630412   0.5630412
[4,]    0.5630412   0.5630412   0.5630412   1.0000000   0.5630412   0.5630412
[5,]    0.5630412   0.5630412   0.5630412   0.5630412   1.0000000   0.5630412
[6,]    0.5630412   0.5630412   0.5630412   0.5630412   0.5630412   1.0000000
```

S-PLUS main programme. Output 12.3 presents a section of the output of a GEE analysis performed with S-PLUS.

The output of S-PLUS is comparable to what has been seen for STATA and SAS. Firstly, some general information is shown (i.e. identity link, Gaussian variance to mean relation and exchangeable correlation structure). Secondly, the results of the analysis are presented. A distinction is made between the 'naive' estimation of the standard errors (which is equal to the 'model-based' estimation procedure) and the 'robust' estimation procedure (both introduced in Section 12.2.1). Finally the scale parameter (i.e. 0.5565875) and the exchangeable correlation (0.5630412) are presented.

The syntax needed to perform a GEE analysis in S-PLUS is as follows:

```
test.gee <- gee(YCONT ~ X1 + X2 + X3 + X4 + TIME,
id=ID, data=long, family=gaussian, corstr="exchangeable")
```

Table 12.1. Summary of the results (i.e. regression coefficients, standard errors (in parentheses), and the scale parameter) of a linear GEE analysis with an exchangeable correlation structure performed with different software packages

	SPIDA[a]	STATA[b]	SAS	S-PLUS
X_1	−0.02 (0.27)	−0.02 (0.28)	−0.03 (0.27)	−0.03 (0.27)
X_2	0.11 (0.02)	0.11 (0.02)	0.11 (0.02)	0.11 (0.02)
X_3	−0.11 (0.06)	−0.11 (0.06)	−0.11 (0.06)	−0.11 (0.06)
X_4	0.10 (0.13)	0.10 (0.12)	0.10 (0.13)	0.10 (0.13)
Time	0.11 (0.01)	0.11 (0.01)	0.11 (0.01)	0.11 (0.01)
Scale parameter	0.75	0.56	0.74	0.56

[a] SPIDA was used in the examples in Chapter 4.
[b] The standard errors estimated in STATA are so-called 'model-based' standard errors; when 'robust' standard errors are calculated the standard errors are exactly the same as for the other packages.

The syntax starts with a typical S-PLUS statement, in which the output of the GEE procedure is linked to an 'object' called test.gee (for details see the S-PLUS manuals). After the GEE procedure specification, the outcome variable and the predictor variables are given. After the comma, additional information has to be specified, i.e. the subject identifier (id=ID), the dataset used (data=long), the distribution of the outcome variable (family= gaussian), and the correlation structure (corstr="exchangeable").

12.2.4 Overview

Table 12.1 summarizes the results of a linear GEE analysis with an exchangeable correlation structure performed with different software packages. From Table 12.1 it can be seen that the results of a GEE analysis with a continuous outcome variable and an exchangeable correlation structure are the same for all four software packages, and although the scale parameters look different, they are also basically the same. With SPIDA and SAS the standard deviation is reported, while STATA and S-PLUS provide the variance.

12.3 GEE analysis with dichotomous outcome variables

12.3.1 STATA

Output 12.4 shows the output of a logistic GEE analysis (i.e. with a dichotomous outcome variable) with an exchangeable correlation structure performed with STATA. The output of the logistic GEE analysis is comparable to Output 12.1, in which the results of the linear GEE analysis were shown. The difference is observed in the 'logit link' and the 'binomial family'. Both indicate that a logistic GEE analysis was performed. Furthermore, it should be noted that (by default) the scale parameter is fixed at a value of one.

Output 12.4. Results of a logistic GEE analysis performed with STATA

```
GEE population-averaged model              Number of obs     =        882
Group variable:                        id  Number of groups  =        147
Link:                               logit  Obs per group: min =         6
Family:                          binomial                avg =        6.0
Correlation:               exchangeable                  max =          6
                                           Wald chi2(5)      =      33.41
Scale parameter:                        1  Prob > chi2       =     0.0000
--------------------------------------------------------------------------
 ydich      Coeff   Std. Err.      z     P > |z|    [95% Conf. Interval]
--------------------------------------------------------------------------
    x1   0.2218124  0.7656789   0.290   0.772   -1.278891    1.722515
    x2   0.3395295  0.0620721   5.470   0.000    0.2178703   0.4611886
    x3  -0.1509501  0.1841475  -0.820   0.412   -0.5118726   0.2099725
    x4   0.0841288  0.336263    0.250   0.802   -0.5749345   0.7431921
  time  -0.0766283  0.0351594  -2.179   0.029   -0.1455396  -0.0077171
 _cons  -2.27018    1.870092   -1.214   0.225   -5.935493    1.395133
```

The syntax needed to perform a logistic GEE analysis in STATA is comparable to that needed to perform a linear GEE analysis, except for the indicators that a dichotomous outcome variable is used (i.e. fam(bin) link(logit)):

```
xtgee ydich x1 x2 x3 x4 time,
i(id) fam(bin) link(logit) corr(exch)
```

Again, the standard errors are, by default, estimated by the 'model-based' procedure. This can be changed by adding 'robust' to the syntax:

```
xtgee ydich x1 x2 x3 x4 time, i(id) fam(bin) link(logit)
corr(exch) robust
```

12.3.2 SAS

Output 12.5 shows a section of the output of a logistic GEE analysis with an exchangeable correlation structure performed with the GENMOD procedure in SAS. It is obvious that the output of a logistic GEE analysis with the GENMOD procedure is comparable to the output of a linear GEE analysis. The difference is the information in the first part of the output, where it is mentioned that a 'logit link' is used with a 'binomial distribution', i.e. that a logistic GEE analysis has been performed. It should be noted that the scale parameter is set at a fixed value of one.

Output 12.5. Results of a logistic GEE analysis performed with the GENMOD procedure in SAS

```
                        The GENMOD Procedure

                         Model Information

Data Set                   LONGBOOK._FIRST_
Distribution                   Binomial
Link Function                   Logit
Dependent Variable              YDICH    DICHOTOMOUS OUTCOME VARIABLE Y
Observations Used                882
Probability Modelled      Pr( YDICH = 1.00 )

                       GEE Model Information

           Correlation Structure          Exchangeable
           Subject Effect             ID (147 levels)
           Number of Clusters                     147
           Correlation Matrix Dimension             6
           Maximum Cluster Size                     6
           Minimum Cluster Size                     6

Algorithm converged

                 Analysis Of GEE Parameter Estimates
                 Empirical Standard Error Estimates

                          Standard     95% Confidence
Parameter    Estimate      Error          Limits              Z      Pr > |Z|
Intercept    -2.2103      1.9173    -5.9681    1.5475      -1.15      0.2490
TIME         -0.0765      0.0372    -0.1494   -0.0036      -2.06      0.0396
X1            0.1964      0.7575    -1.2882    1.6811       0.26      0.7954
X2            0.3392      0.0627     0.2163    0.4620       5.41     <0.0001
X3           -0.1514      0.1979    -0.5392    0.2364      -0.77      0.4442
X4            0.0784      0.3741    -0.6547    0.8116       0.21      0.8339
```

The syntax needed to perform a logistic GEE analysis with the GENMOD procedure is comparable to that discussed for the linear GEE analysis. The only difference is found in the third line, where it has to be specified that the outcome variable is dichotomous (link=logit and dist=binomial):

```
proc genmod data=long.x;
class id;
model ydich = x1 x2 x3 x4 time /link=logit dist=binomial;
repeated subject=id/type=exch;
run;
```

12.3.3 S-PLUS

Output 12.6 shows a section of the result of a logistic GEE analysis with an exchangeable correlation structure performed with S-PLUS. As for STATA and SAS, the output of a logistic GEE analysis performed with S-PLUS is comparable to that discussed for a linear GEE analysis. Again, the only difference

Output 12.6. Results of a logistic GEE analysis performed with S-PLUS

```
Model:
 Link:                        Logit
 Variance to Mean Relation: Binomial
 Correlation Structure:      Exchangeable

Coefficients:
               Estimate   Naive S.E.     Naive z   Robust S.E.    Robust z
(Intercept)  -2.21034233  1.83678846  -1.2033734   1.91727343  -1.1528571
        X1    0.19645777  0.75221479   0.2611724   0.75750897   0.2593471
        X2    0.33915553  0.06094529   5.5649181   0.06265946   5.4126786
        X3   -0.15140556  0.18079601  -0.8374386   0.19786875  -0.7651818
        X4    0.07842177  0.33027236   0.2374457   0.37406819   0.2096456
      TIME   -0.07652509  0.03452004  -2.2168307   0.03718649  -2.0578735

Estimated Scale Parameter: 0.9642425
Number of Iterations: 4

Working Correlation
            [,1]        [,2]        [,3]        [,4]        [,5]        [,6]
[1,]   1.0000000   0.4884038   0.4884038   0.4884038   0.4884038   0.4884038
[2,]   0.4884038   1.0000000   0.4884038   0.4884038   0.4884038   0.4884038
[3,]   0.4884038   0.4884038   1.0000000   0.4884038   0.4884038   0.4884038
[4,]   0.4884038   0.4884038   0.4884038   1.0000000   0.4884038   0.4884038
[5,]   0.4884038   0.4884038   0.4884038   0.4884038   1.0000000   0.4884038
[6,]   0.4884038   0.4884038   0.4884038   0.4884038   0.4884038   1.0000000
```

Table 12.2. Summary of the results (i.e. regression coefficients, standard errors (in parentheses), and the scale parameter) of a logistic GEE analysis with an exchangeable correlation structure performed with different software packages

	SPIDA[a]	STATA[b]	SAS	S-PLUS
X_1	0.22 (0.76)	0.22 (0.77)	0.20 (0.76)	0.20 (0.76)
X_2	0.34 (0.06)	0.34 (0.06)	0.34 (0.06)	0.34 (0.06)
X_3	−0.15 (0.20)	−0.15 (0.18)	−0.15 (0.20)	−0.15 (0.20)
X_4	0.08 (0.37)	0.08 (0.34)	0.08 (0.37)	0.08 (0.37)
Time	−0.08 (0.04)	−0.08 (0.04)	−0.08 (0.04)	−0.08 (0.04)
Scale parameter	0.98	1	1	0.96

[a] SPIDA was used in the examples in Chapter 6.
[b] The standard errors estimated in STATA are so-called 'model based' standard errors; when 'robust' standard errors are calculated the standard errors are exactly the same as for the other packages.

is found in the 'logit link' and the 'binomial variance to mean relation'. The syntax needed to obtain a logistic GEE analysis is also fairly straightforward:

```
test.gee <- gee(YDICH ~ X1 + X2 + X3 + X4 + TIME, id=ID,
data=long, family=binomial, corstr="exchangeable")
```

12.3.4 Overview

Table 12.2 summarizes the results of the logistic GEE analysis with an exchangeable correlation structure performed with different software packages. As was the case with the linear GEE analysis, the results obtained from the logistic GEE analysis with different software packages are almost the same.

12.4 Random coefficient analysis with continuous outcome variables

12.4.1 STATA

STATA was used in the examples in Chapter 4, so the output will not be repeated here. The analyses discussed in that chapter were performed with two different procedures. The **xtreg** procedure is suitable for performing a linear random coefficient analysis with only a random intercept, whereas the 'generalized linear latent and mixed models' (GLLAMM) procedure can be used when more than one random coefficient has to be estimated (Rabe-Hesketh et al., 2001a, 2001b). This procedure is not available in the standard software, but it can easily be implemented. One major disadvantage of the GLLAMM procedure is that the time needed to estimate the regression coefficients is extremely long. The syntax of the **xtreg** procedure is highly comparable to the syntax of the **xtgee** procedure:

```
xtreg ycont x1 x2 x3 x4 time, i(id)
```

The syntax of the GLLAMM procedure is slightly more extensive:

```
gen con=1
eq int:con
eq slope:time
gllamm ycont x1 x2 x3 x4 time, i(id) nrf(2) eqs
(int slope) nip(12)
```

The first line of the syntax for the GLLAMM procedure is needed to define a row of ones, which is necessary to define the random intercept (eq int:con). Furthermore the random slope with time is defined (eq slope:time). The GLLAMM procedure is then the same as all other STATA commands. After the procedure specification, the outcome variable is directly followed by the predictor variables, and after the comma additional information is provided, i.e. the subject identifier (i(id)), the number of random coefficients (nrf(2)), and the definition of the random coefficients (eqs(int slope)). 'Nip' stands for the number of integration points, which are used to estimate the likelihood of the random coefficient analysis. It goes far beyond the scope of this book to explain this estimation procedure in detail. Detailed information can be found in the software manual (Rabe-Hesketh et al., 2001a), and in several publications (Rabe-Hesketh and Pickles, 1999; Rabe-Hesketh et al., 2000, 2001b).

12.4.2 SAS

Within SAS, the MIXED procedure can be used to perform linear random coefficient analysis (i.e. with a continuous outcome variable). Output 12.7

Output 12.7. Results of a linear random coefficient analysis with only a random intercept performed with the MIXED procedure in SAS

```
                    The Mixed Procedure
                    Model Information

Data Set                        LONGBOOK._FIRST_
Dependent Variable              YCONT
Covariance Structure            Unstructured
Subject Effect                  ID
Estimation Method               REML
Residual Variance Method        Profile
Fixed Effects SE Method         Model-Based
Degrees of Freedom Method       Containment

                        Dimensions
            Covariance Parameters        2
            Columns in X                 6
            Columns in Z Per Subject     1
            Subjects                   147
            Max Obs Per Subject          6
            Observations Used          882
            Observations Not Used        0
            Total Observations         882

                Covariance Parameter Estimates
            Cov Parm      Subject    Estimate
            UN(1,1)        ID          0.3205
            Residual                   0.2412

                        Fit Statistics
            Res Log Likelihood                -795.0
            Akaike's Information Criterion    -797.0
            Schwarz's Bayesian Criterion      -800.0
            -2 Res Log Likelihood             1590.1

                    Solution for Fixed Effects
                            Standard
Effect       Estimate       Error      DF    t Value    Pr > |t|

Intercept     3.6378        0.6786     144     5.36      <0.0001
TIME          0.1077        0.01106    732     9.74      <0.0001
X1           -0.03122       0.2784     732    -0.11       0.9108
X2            0.1102        0.02004    732     5.50      <0.0001
X3           -0.1140        0.05812    732    -1.96       0.0502
X4            0.09957       0.1226     732     0.81       0.4170
```

shows the results of a linear random coefficient analysis with only a random intercept performed with the MIXED procedure in SAS. Because the length of the original output is quite large, only a section of the output is shown.

A few important messages can be derived from Output 12.7. First of all, it is shown that the method of estimation is restricted maximum likelihood (REML). In Chapter 4 it has already been mentioned that there is some debate about the use of either a maximum likelihood or restricted maximum likelihood estimation method. Both methods are available with the MIXED procedure in SAS, but because restricted maximum likelihood is the default procedure, these results have been reported. The next part of the output, which is of interest, is where the covariance parameter estimates are presented. UN(1,1) is the variance of the normally distributed random intercept, and 'residual' is the error variance.

In addition to the variance parameters, some fit statistics are also provided. Because REML was used, the -2 res log likelihood was estimated instead of the -2 log likelihood. The interpretation is, however, basically the same. Furthermore, Akaike's information criterion and Schwarz's Bayesian criterion are presented. Both can be seen as 'adjusted' values of the -2 (res) log likelihood, i.e. adjusted for the number of parameters estimated by the particular model (Akaike, 1974; Schwarz, 1978).

The last part of the output shows the estimates of the regression coefficients, the standard errors, the degrees of freedom, the t-values (derived from the regression coefficient divided by the standard error) and the corresponding p-values. It should be noted that in the MIXED procedure the t-distribution is used instead of the standard normal distribution (z-distribution), which is used in STATA. Using the t-distribution leads to slightly higher p-values, especially when the number of observations is low.

Output 12.8 shows (a section of) the output of a linear random coefficient analysis with both a random intercept and a random slope with time. The most important difference between Output 12.7 and Output 12.8 is the number of covariance parameters that are estimated. In the analysis with both a random intercept and a random slope with time, three covariance parameters are estimated: (1) UN(1,1) which is an estimate of the standard deviation of the normally distributed random intercept, (2) UN(2,2) which is an estimate of the standard deviation of the normally distributed random slope with time, and (3) UN(1,2) which is an estimate of the covariance between the random intercept and the random slope. Furthermore, the value

Output 12.8. Results of a linear random coefficient analysis with a random intercept and a random slope with time performed with the MIXED procedure in SAS

The Mixed Procedure

Model Information

Data Set	LONGBOOK._FIRST_
Dependent Variable	YCONT
Covariance Structure	Unstructured
Subject Effect	ID
Estimation Method	REML
Residual Variance Method	Profile
Fixed Effects SE Method	Model-Based
Degrees of Freedom Method	Containment

Dimensions

Covariance Parameters	4
Columns in X	6
Columns in Z Per Subject	2
Subjects	147
Max Obs Per Subject	6
Observations Used	882
Observations Not Used	0
Total Observations	882

Covariance Parameter Estimates

Cov Parm	Subject	Estimate
UN(1,1)	ID	0.2731
UN(2,1)	ID	-0.00120
UN(2,2)	ID	0.004955
Residual		0.2238

Fit Statistics

Res Log Likelihood	-788.9
Akaike's Information Criterion	-792.9
Schwarz's Bayesian Criterion	-798.9
-2 Res Log Likelihood	1577.8

Solution for Fixed Effects

Effect	Estimate	Standard Error	DF	t Value	Pr > |t|
Intercept	3.7102	0.6682	144	5.55	<0.0001
TIME	0.1090	0.01224	146	8.91	<0.0001
X1	-0.01986	0.2740	586	-0.07	0.9423
X2	0.1069	0.02038	586	5.24	<0.0001
X3	-0.1239	0.05950	586	-2.08	0.0377
X4	0.04386	0.1202	586	0.36	0.7152

of the -2 res log likelihood is different. The difference between the -2 res log likelihoods can be used to evaluate the necessity of the random slope with time. The difference is 12.3, which follows a χ^2 distribution with two degrees of freedom (i.e. the variance of the random slope with time and the covariance between the random intercept and slope), which is highly significant.

The syntax needed to perform a linear random coefficient analysis with both a random intercept and a random slope with time is shown below:

```
proc mixed data=long.x;
class id;
model ycont = x1 x2 x3 x4 time/s;
random int time/ subject=id;
run;
```

The syntax looks similar to that needed to perform a GEE analysis with the GENMOD procedure. The difference is firstly that the 'repeated' statement is replaced by the 'random' statement, which is necessary in order to identify the random coefficients (i.e. intercept (int) and time). Secondly there is no specification of the correlation structure needed.

12.4.3 S-PLUS

Within S-PLUS, linear random coefficient analysis is referred to as 'linear mixed effects model'. Output 12.9 shows the result of a linear random coefficient analysis with only a random intercept. The first line of the output shows that the parameters of this linear mixed effects model were estimated with restricted maximum likelihood (REML). As with the MIXED procedure in SAS, the REML estimation procedure is default, although it is also possible to perform a maximum likelihood estimation procedure. In the same block of the output, the log likelihood of the model is shown, in addition to some other fit measures. AIC and BIC stand, respectively, for Akaike's information criterion and Schwarz's Bayesian criterion.

The next part of the output shows the random effects. In a model with only a random intercept, two variance parameters are estimated (given as standard deviations in the S-PLUS output): the standard deviation of the normally distributed random intercept (0.5661159) and the residual (or error) standard deviation (0.491077). The following part of the output shows the estimates of the regression coefficients, the standard errors of the regression coefficients, the degrees of freedom, the t-values (i.e. the regression coefficient divided by its standard error), and the corresponding p-values. Note that

Output 12.9. Results of a linear random coefficient analysis with only a random intercept performed with S-PLUS

```
Linear Mixed Effects Model
Linear mixed-effects model fit by REML
 Data: longlang
       AIC       BIC       logLik
  1606.062  1644.265   -795.0312

Random effects:
 Formula: ~ 1 | ID
          (Intercept)      Residual
StdDev:   0.5661159        0.491077
Fixed effects: YCONT    ~ X1 + X2 + X3 + X4 + TIME
                  Value    Std.Error    DF     t-value    p-value
(Intercept)     3.637756   0.6786008   732    5.360672   <0.0001
        X1     -0.031219   0.2784197   144   -0.112129    0.9109
        X2      0.110187   0.0200419   732    5.497859   <0.0001
        X3     -0.113991   0.0581185   732   -1.961354    0.0502
        X4      0.099572   0.1226030   144    0.812152    0.4180
      TIME      0.107736   0.0110569   732    9.743772   <0.0001

Number of Observations: 882
Number of Groups: 147
```

also with S-PLUS, the t-distribution is used instead of the standard normal distribution.

Output 12.10 shows the results of a linear random coefficient analysis with both a random intercept and a random slope with time performed with S-PLUS. It is obvious that the most important difference between Output 12.9 and Output 12.10 is the estimation of two more random effects, i.e. the random slope with time and the correlation between the random intercept and the random slope. As in all the other types of random coefficient analysis, the necessity of the random slope with time can be estimated with the likelihood ratio test. The difference between the -2 log likelihood of the analysis with only a random intercept and the -2 log likelihood of the analysis with both a random intercept and a random slope is exactly the same as was calculated with the MIXED procedure in SAS, i.e. 12.3.

With S-PLUS, the 'linear mixed effects model' is implemented in the menu-driven standard software package, so no syntax is needed to perform a linear random coefficient analysis.

Output 12.10. Results of a random coefficient analysis with a random intercept and a random slope with time performed with S-PLUS

```
Linear mixed-effects model fit by REML
 Data: longbook
       AIC        BIC      logLik
  1597.817   1645.571   -788.9087

Random effects:
 Formula:  ~ TIME | ID
 Structure: General positive-definite
             StdDev        Corr
(Intercept) 0.52225722   (Inter
       TIME 0.07030164    -0.03
   Residual 0.47310997

Fixed effects: YCONT    ~ X1 + X2 + X3 + X4 + TIME
              Value    Std.Error    DF    t-value    p-value
(Intercept)  3.710474  0.6681977   732   5.552958   <0.0001
        X1  -0.019858  0.2740515   144  -0.072462    0.9423
        X2   0.106854  0.0203809   732   5.242826   <0.0001
        X3  -0.123972  0.0595020   732  -2.083497    0.0376
        X4   0.043717  0.1201785   144   0.363766    0.7166
      TIME   0.109037  0.0122370   732   8.910435   <0.0001

Number of Observations: 882
Number of Groups: 147
```

12.4.4 SPSS

Before the release of version 11, with SPSS it was not possible to perform sophisticated longitudinal data analysis. However, in version 11, random coefficient analysis for continuous outcome variables became available. This new procedure, which is based on the algorithms discussed by Wolfinger et al. (1994) can be derived from the menu and is called 'mixed models – linear'. Output 12.11 shows a section of the output of a random coefficient analysis with only a random intercept performed in SPSS. The first part of the output shows the information criteria. First of all the −2 restricted log likelihood is provided (1590.062). This indicates that restricted maximum likelihood is used as default estimation procedure. Besides the −2 restricted log likelihood, values of other fit measures are also shown. AIC and BIC were also provided by other software packages and can be seen as 'adjusted' values

Output 12.11. Results of a linear random coefficient analysis with only a random intercept performed with SPSS

Information criteria[a]

-2 Restricted Log Likelihood	1590.062
Akaike's Information Criterion (AIC)	1594.062
Hurvich and Tsai's Criterion (AICC)	1594.076
Bozdogan's Criterion (CAIC)	1605.613
Schwarz's Bayesian Criterion (BIC)	1603.613

The information criteria are displayed in smaller-is-better forms.

[a]Dependent Variable: OUTCOME VARIABLE Y.

Estimates of fixed effects[a]

						95% Confidence Interval	
Parameter	Estimate	Std. Error	df	t	Sig	Lower Bound	Upper Bound
Intercept	3.6377560	0.6786008	148.384	5.361	0.000	2.2967864	4.9787257
X1	-3.1×10^{-2}	0.2784197	146.529	-0.112	0.911	0.5814559	0.5190181
X2	0.1101875	2.00×10^{-2}	875.829	5.498	0.000	7.085174×10^{-2}	0.1495232
X3	0.1139909	5.81×10^{-2}	829.228	-1.961	0.050	-0.2280675	8.573713×10^{-5}
X4	9.96×10^{-2}	0.1226030	148.710	0.812	0.418	-0.1426967	0.3418412
TIME	0.1077357	1.11×10^{-2}	775.479	9.744	0.000	8.603073×10^{-2}	0.1294406

[a]Dependent Variable: OUTCOME VARIABLE Y.

Estimate of covariance parameters[a]

Parameter		Estimate	Std. Error
Repeated Measures	CS diagonal offset	0.2411566	1.26×10^{-2}
	CS covariance	0.32045872	4.29×10^{-2}

[a]Dependent Variable: OUTCOME VARIABLE Y.

of the -2 restricted log likelihood. Hurvich and Tsai's criterion (AICC) and Bozdogan's criterion (CAIC) are slightly different but can be interpreted in more or less the same way (Bozdogan, 1987; Hurvich and Tsai, 1989). The next part of the output shows the estimates of fixed effects. In this part of the output, the regression coefficients, the standard errors, the degrees of freedom, the t-values, the corresponding p-values, and the 95% confidence interval around the regression coefficient are provided. The last part of the output shows the estimates of covariance parameters. Because only a random intercept was allowed in the analysis, only the variance of the normally distributed random intercept (0.3204872) and the remaining error variance (0.2411566) are provided.

Output 12.12 shows (a section of) the output of a random coefficient analysis with both a random intercept and a random slope with time performed with SPSS. The output looks similar to the one discussed for the analysis with only a random intercept. The difference is found in the last part in which the estimates of covariance parameters are given. Besides the variance of the random intercept and the remaining error variance, the random variance of the slope with time is also given (i.e. 4.76×10^{-3}). Similar to all other random coefficient analyses, with the -2 restricted log likelihood values of the two analyses discussed, the necessity of allowing a random slope with time can be evaluated.

12.4.5 MLwiN

Multilevel analysis for windows (MLwiN) is specifically developed to perform random coefficient analysis. Output 12.13 shows the results of a linear random coefficient analysis with only a random intercept. Because MLwiN is specifically developed to perform multilevel analysis, the levels of the analysis must first be defined. In the case of longitudinal data, the observations over time are nested within subjects so, in this special case, time is the lowest level of analysis and subject is the highest level of analysis. It should be noted that in the MLwiN output the lowest level (time) is indicated by the subscript i, and the highest level (subject) is indicated by the subscript j. This is different from the regular notation, in which subjects are usually indicated by the subscript i.

The first line of the output shows that the outcome variable Y is a continuous normally distributed variable. In the second line the model is given,

Output 12.12. Results of a linear random coefficient analysis with a random intercept and a random slope with time performed with SPSS

Information criteria[a]

-2 Restricted Log Likelihood	1577.835
Akaike's Information Criterion (AIC)	1583.835
Hurvich and Tsai's Criterion (AICC)	1583.862
Bozdogan's Criterion (CAIC)	1601.161
Schwarz's Bayesian Criterion (BIC)	1598.161

The information criteria are displayed in smaller-is-better forms.

[a]Dependent Variable: OUTCOME VARIABLE Y.

Estimates of fixed effects[a]

						95% Confidence Interval	
Parameter	Estimate	Std. Error	df	t	Sig	Lower Bound	Upper Bound
Intercept	3.7145121	0.6683017	117.755	5.558	0.000	2.3910643	5.0379600
X1	-2.0×10^{-2}	0.2740982	116.508	-0.072	0.942	-0.5626915	0.5230306
X2	0.1065286	2.04×10^{-2}	500.682	5.231	0.000	6.651527×10^{-2}	0.1465419
X3	-0.1244969	5.95×10^{-2}	494.624	-2.092	0.037	-0.2413992	-7.5946×10^{-3}
X4	4.17×10^{-2}	0.1201765	118.409	0.347	0.729	-0.1963073	0.2796401
TIME	0.1091382	1.22×10^{-2}	203.227	8.950	0.000	8.509509×10^{-2}	0.1331814

[a]Dependent Variable: OUTCOME VARIABLE Y.

Estimates of covariance parameters[a]

Parameter		Estimate	Std. Error
Repeated Measures	CS diagonal offset	0.2243005	1.26×10^{-2}
	CS covariance	0.2681568	4.24×10^{-2}
TIME [subject = ID]	ID diagonal	4.76×10^{-3}	1.66×10^{-3}

[a]Dependent Variable: OUTCOME VARIABLE Y.

Output 12.13. Results of a linear random coefficient analysis with only a random intercept performed with MLwiN

```
ycont_ij ~ N(XB, Ω)
ycont_ij = β_0ij cons + 0.109(0.011)time_ij + -0.024(0.276) x 1_j +
0.111(0.020) x 2_ij + -0.111(0.058) x 3_ij + 0.101(0.121) x 4_j
β_0ij = 3.617(0.672) + u_0j + e_0ij
[u_0j] ~ N(0, Ω_u) : Ω_u = [0.313(0.041)]
[e_0ij] ~ N(0, Ω_e) : Ω_e = [0.242(0.013)]
-2*log(like) = 1569.928
```

with the intercept β_0 ('cons' stands for a row of ones, which has no meaning, but is necessary for the estimation of the intercept), the fixed regression coefficient for time (0.109 with standard error 0.011), and the fixed regression coefficients for the four predictor variables (X_1 to X_4). The regression coefficients can be tested for significance by dividing the coefficient by its standard error. As in GEE analysis, this ratio is known as the Wald statistic, which approximately follows a standard normal distribution. Furthermore, from the output it can be seen that X_1 and X_4 are time-independent predictor variables (subscript j, so only varying between subjects), X_2 and X_3 are time-dependent predictor variables (subscript ij, so varying between time-points and between subjects).

The third line of the output provides information about the random intercept β_0. The coefficient consists of a fixed part (3.617 with standard error 0.672) and an error variance which is divided into two parts: the first part μ is the random variation in the intercept and the second part ε is the total 'error' variance. In the next two lines these variances are given, with the corresponding standard errors ($\mu = 0.313$ (0.041) and $\varepsilon = 0.242$ (0.013)).

The last line of the output presents the -2 log likelihood (1569.928) which can be used in comparison with the -2 log likelihood from a model with both a random intercept and a random slope with time (see Output 12.14).

From Output 12.14 it can be seen that in addition to a random intercept, a random slope is considered. For the regression coefficient for time (β_1) a within-subject variation μ is considered (fourth line in the output). So three variance parameters are estimated: the random variation of the intercept (0.263 with standard error 0.055), the random variation of the slope with time (0.005 with standard error 0.002), and the covariance between random intercept and slope (0.000 with standard error 0.009).

Output 12.14. Results of a linear random coefficient analysis with a random intercept and a random slope with time performed with MLwiN

$$\text{ycont}_{ij} \sim \text{N}(XB, \ \Omega)$$

$\text{ycont}_{ij} = \beta_{0ij}\text{cons} + \beta_{1j}\text{time}_{ij} + -0.013(0.271) \ \text{x} \ 1_j + 0.170(0.020)$
$\qquad \text{x} \ 2_{ij} + -0.121(0.060) \ \text{x} \ 3_{ij} + 0.044(0.119) \ \text{x} \ 4_j$

$\beta_{0ij} = 3.694(0.661) + u_{0j} + e_{0ij}$
$\beta_{1j} = 0.110(0.012) + u_{1j}$

$$\begin{bmatrix} u_{0j} \\ u_{1j} \end{bmatrix} \sim \text{N}(0, \ \Omega_u) \ : \ \Omega_u = \begin{bmatrix} 0.263(0.055) & \\ 0.000(0.009) & 0.005(0.002) \end{bmatrix}$$

$[e_{0ij}] \sim \text{N}(0, \ \Omega_e) \ : \ \Omega_e = [0.225(0.013)]$

$-2*\log(\text{like}) = 1557.898$

The likelihood ratio test can be used to decide whether or not a random slope should be added to the model. The difference between the -2 log likelihood of the model without a random slope (i.e. 1569.928) and a model with a random slope with time (i.e. 1557.898)) is 12.03, which follows a χ^2 distribution with two degrees of freedom, and is highly significant. It should be noted that the log likelihood values obtained from MLwiN are slightly different to those obtained from SAS and S-PLUS. This is due to the fact that with MLwiN an iterative generalized least squares (IGLS) approach is used by default, which is basically the same as maximum likelihood, and that with SAS and S-PLUS restricted maximum likelihood is used. With MLwiN a so-called restricted iterative generalized least squares (RIGLS) estimation procedure can also be used, which is comparable to restricted maximum likelihood (Goldstein, 1986, 1989, 1995). Because with MLwiN the random coefficient analysis can be directly derived from the menu, no syntax is needed.

12.4.6 Overview

Table 12.3 summarizes the results of the linear random coefficient analyses with both a random intercept and a random slope with time performed with different software packages. From Table 12.3 it can be seen that using a different software package does not lead to different results of the linear random coefficient analysis. This is irrespective of the estimation procedure used, because the results derived from SAS, S-PLUS, or SPSS (i.e. all packages use the REML estimation procedure as default) did not differ from the results derived from STATA and MLwiN (i.e. both packages use the maximum likelihood estimation procedure). It is often argued that the REML approach

Table 12.3. Summary of the results (i.e. regression coefficients, standard errors (in parentheses), −2 log likelihoods and random variances) of a linear random coefficient analysis with both a random intercept and a random slope with time performed with different software packages

	STATA[a]	SAS[b]	MLwiN[a]	S-PLUS[b]	SPSS[b]
X_1	−0.02 (0.27)	−0.02 (0.27)	−0.01 (0.27)	−0.02 (0.27)	−0.02 (0.27)
X_2	0.11 (0.02)	0.11 (0.02)	0.11 (0.02)	0.11 (0.02)	0.11 (0.02)
X_3	−0.12 (0.06)	−0.12 (0.06)	−0.12 (0.06)	−0.12 (0.06)	−0.12 (0.06)
X_4	0.04 (0.12)	0.04 (0.12)	0.04 (0.12)	0.04 (0.12)	0.04 (0.12)
Time	0.11 (0.01)	0.11 (0.01)	0.11 (0.01)	0.11 (0.01)	0.11 (0.01)
−2 log likelihood	1557.8	1577.8	1557.9	1577.8	1577.8
Random variance					
Intercept	0.265	0.273	0.263	0.273[c]	0.268
Slope	0.005	0.005	0.005	0.005[c]	0.005

[a] Estimated with maximum likelihood.
[b] Estimated with restricted maximum likelihood.
[c] In the original output standard deviations are given.

gives a 'better' estimation of the variance components in the random coefficient analysis. However, although there is a difference in the variance of the intercept, this difference is very small and does not affect the magnitude of the regression coefficients or the standard errors of the regression coefficients.

12.5 Random coefficient analysis with dichotomous outcome variables

12.5.1 Introduction

In Chapter 6 it has already been mentioned that logistic random coefficient analysis (i.e. with dichotomous outcome variables) is quite difficult to perform. Basically there are two possible approaches. The most straightforward approach is the Gauss–Hermite technique, which is based on Gaussian quadrature points (see also Section 12.4.1). The second approach is based on so-called penalized quasi-likelihood (PQL). However, it is far beyond the scope of this book to explain these techniques in detail. For more information, reference is made to the more technical literature (e.g. Goldstein, 1991; Schall, 1991; Breslow and Clayton, 1993; Longford, 1993; Liu and

Pierce, 1994; Pinheiro and Bates, 1995; Goldstein and Rasbash, 1996; Agresti et al., 2000; Lesaffre and Spiessens, 2001), and the reference manuals of the different software packages. Because of the estimation problems, not all software packages provide facilities to perform a logistic random coefficient analysis. With STATA and SAS, the Gauss–Hermite technique is available, while in MLwiN the PQL procedure can be applied. Unfortunately, a procedure for logistic random coefficient analysis has not yet been developed in S-PLUS.

12.5.2 STATA

In the examples discussed in Chapter 6, STATA was used to perform a logistic random coefficient analysis. It should be noted that in the standard STATA software, random coefficient analysis can only be performed with **one** random coefficient (e.g. a random intercept). This is implemented in the **xtlogit** procedure. The syntax needed for this procedure is as follows:

```
xtlogit ydich x1 x2 x3 x4 time, i(id) fam(bin) link(logit)
```

For random coefficient analysis with more random regression coefficients, the GLLAMM procedure can be used:

```
gen con=1
eq int:con
eq slope:time
gllamm ydich x1 x2 x3 x4 time,
i(id) fam(bin) link(logit) nrf(2) eqs(int slope) nip(12)
```

The syntax for both procedures is comparable to the syntax described for the linear random coefficient analysis. In the syntax for the logistic random coefficient analysis additionally the binomial family and the logit link have to be specified.

In the examples presented in Chapter 6, the GLLAMM procedure was used with 12 quadrature points. Unfortunately, in contrast to linear random coefficient analysis, the results of logistic random coefficient analysis highly depend on the number of quadrature points used in the estimation procedure. To illustrate this, Table 12.4 gives a summary of the results of several logistic random coefficient analyses with a different number of quadrature points.

The results summarized in Table 12.4 are very clear. Although the analysis is quite simple (i.e. only a random intercept and a random slope with

Table 12.4. Summary of the results (i.e. regression coefficients and standard errors (in parentheses), and random variances) of logistic random coefficient analyses with a different number of quadrature points

	Number of quadrature points			
	4	10	12	15
X_1	0.26 (1.36)	0.43 (1.57)	0.33 (1.63)	0.15 (1.22)
X_2	0.75 (0.14)	0.73 (0.14)	0.72 (0.14)	0.73 (0.13)
X_3	−0.15 (0.41)	−0.23 (0.36)	−0.23 (0.36)	−0.14 (0.34)
X_4	0.26 (0.54)	0.44 (0.66)	0.46 (0.70)	0.23 (0.55)
Time	−0.17 (0.09)	−0.08 (0.09)	−0.07 (0.10)	−0.02 (0.10)
Random variance				
Intercept	9.639	12.519	13.116	18.064
Slope	0.114	0.107	0.109	0.165

time, and only four predictor variables and time), the results of the analyses differ remarkably. This was also recognized by other authors who carried out similar comparisons (e.g. Lesaffre and Spiessens, 2001). In the statistical literature, it is generally accepted that 10 quadrature points are sufficient for a 'valid' logistic random coefficient analysis, although others suggest that 20 quadrature points are needed (e.g. Hu et al., 1998; Rodriguez and Goldman, 2001). However, in the present example, as well as in examples presented by others (e.g. Lesaffre and Spiessens, 2001), neither of these suggestions is confirmed.

12.5.3 SAS

A few years ago, a SAS macro called GLIMMIX that can be used to perform logistic random coefficient analysis became available (Breslow and Clayton, 1993). However, the performance of this procedure was not very satisfactory (Wolfinger, 1998; Lesaffre and Spiessens, 2001). Basically, GLIMMIX is only suitable when the number of observations per subject is fairly large; unfortunately, in the field of epidemiological research this is almost never the case. Nowadays the NLMIXED procedure is available for logistic random coefficient analysis. Output 12.15 shows (a section of) the results of a logistic random coefficient analysis with both a random intercept and a random slope with time performed with the NLMIXED procedure in SAS.

Output 12.15. Results of a logistic random coefficient analysis with both a random intercept and a random slope with time performed with the NLMIXED procedure in SAS

```
                    The NLMIXED Procedure

                       Specifications

Description                               Value

Data Set                                  WORK.LONG
Dependent Variable                        YDICH
Distribution for Dependent Variable       Binary
Random Effects                            b0 b1
Distribution for Random Effects           Normal
Subject Variable                          ID
Optimization Technique                    Dual Quasi-Newton
Integration Method                        Adaptive Gaussian
                                          Quadrature

                         Dimensions

Description                               Value

Observations Used                         882
Observations Not Used                     0
Total Observations                        882
Subjects                                  147
Max Obs Per Subject                       6
Parameters                                9
Quadrature Points                         9
```

Parameters

beta0	beta1	beta2	beta3	beta4	beta5	s2b0	s2b1	cb01
-4	-1	0.4	0.7	-0.2	0.4	12	0.1	-1

Parameters

NOTE: GCONV convergence criterion satisfied.

Fit Statistics

Description	Value
-2 Log Likelihood	793.8
AIC (smaller is better)	811.8
BIC (smaller is better)	838.7
Log Likelihood	-396.9
AIC (larger is better)	-405.9
BIC (larger is better)	-419.3

The NLMIXED Procedure

Parameter Estimates

Parameter	Estimate	Standard Error	DF	t Value	Pr > |t|	Alpha	Lower	Upper	Gradient
beta0	-4.9683	3.4950	145	-1.42	0.1573	0.05	-11.8761	1.9395	0.000447
beta1	-0.03663	0.09878	145	-0.37	0.7113	0.05	-0.2319	0.1586	0.001249
beta2	0.1546	1.4308	145	0.11	0.9141	0.05	-2.6733	2.9824	0.000912
beta3	0.7156	0.1337	145	5.35	<0.0001	0.05	0.4513	0.9799	0.001093
beta4	-0.1904	0.3492	145	-0.55	0.5864	0.05	-0.8805	0.4997	0.000031
beta5	0.3275	0.6253	145	0.52	0.6013	0.05	-0.9085	1.5634	0.000677
s2b0	15.9054	5.7868	145	2.75	0.0067	0.05	4.4681	27.3428	0.000063
s2b1	0.1380	0.1136	145	1.21	0.2265	0.05	-0.08654	0.3624	-0.00044
cb01	-1.3636	0.8053	145	-1.69	0.0925	0.05	-2.95517668	-0.00234	

The output of the NLMIXED procedure is not very straightforward, and deserves further explanation. The first part of the output provides general information about the estimation procedure. It can be seen that a binary outcome variable is used (i.e. that a logistic random coefficient analysis has been performed) and that there are two random effects, which are both normally distributed. Furthermore, it shows that a dual quasi-Newton algorithm is used and that an adaptive Gaussian quadrature method is used. The latter can be seen as an extension to the standard Gauss–Hermite technique (for details, see for instance Lesaffre and Spiessens, 2001). The dual quasi-Newton algorithm is one of the possible optimization techniques available for logistic random coefficient analysis which will not be discussed any further (for details see the software manuals). From the next part of the output it can be seen that nine quadrature points are used for the estimation (by default the NLMIXED procedure in SAS defines more or less by itself how many quadrature points are needed, although it can be changed manually). It also shows that nine parameters are estimated, the starting values of which are shown below the general information. The problems with the NLMIXED procedure in SAS are that the user has to provide the starting values for the different parameters and (even more problematic) that the final results of the estimated regression coefficients and standard errors can depend on the choice of these starting values. If no starting values are provided, the NLMIXED procedure assumes a starting value of one for all parameters. The nine parameters to be estimated correspond with the intercept (beta0), the regression coefficient for time (beta1), the regression coefficients for the four predictor variables X_1 to X_4 (beta2 to beta5), the random variance of the intercept (s2b0), the random variance of the slope with time (s2b1), and the covariance (interaction) between the random intercept and the random slope with time (cb01).

The next part of the output shows the results: firstly the fit of the model (i.e. the (-2) log likelihood, Akaike's information criterion, and Schwarz's Bayesian criterion), and secondly the information regarding the regression coefficients and the random components, including standard errors, 95% confidence intervals, and p-values (which are based on the t-distribution). The most important parts of the output are the regression coefficients, the corresponding standard errors and the variances of the random coefficients.

The syntax needed to perform a logistic random coefficient analysis with the NLMIXED procedure is rather complicated:

```
proc nlmixed data=long;
parms beta0=-4 beta1=-1 beta2=0.6 beta3 =1 beta4=
-1 beta5=1 s2b0=6 s2b1=1 cb01=1;
c1 = beta0 + b0;
c2 = beta1 + b1;
eta = c1 + (c2*time)+ beta2*x1 + beta3*x2 + beta4*x3
+ beta5*x4;
expeta = exp(eta);
p = expeta / (1+expeta);
model ydich ~ binary(p);
random b0 b1 ~ normal([0,0],[s2b0,cb01,s2b1]) subject=id;
run;
```

With the 'parms' statement, starting values are assigned to all parameters that are to be estimated. After this, the random coefficients are specified for the intercept (c1) and for the slope with time (c2). In the next lines the logistic model is specified, while in the last line of this command the random effects are defined.

12.5.4 MLwiN

Output 12.16 shows the results of a logistic random coefficient analysis with both a random intercept and a random slope with time performed with MLwiN. The MLwiN output with a dichotomous outcome variable is similar to the MLwiN output with a continuous outcome variable. The first line of the output shows that a binomial distribution is used (i.e. that a dichotomous outcome variable is analysed). 'Denom' and 'bcons' are specifications for (generally) rows of ones, which are needed to perform the logistic random coefficient analysis (for details see the software manual). The next part of the output shows that the logit is analysed, which indicates that a logistic random coefficient analysis has been performed, and provides the regression coefficients and the standard errors, which can be evaluated in exactly the same way as has been described for a linear random coefficient analysis performed with MLwiN. Furthermore, information about the random part of the analysis is given: the variance of the normally distributed random intercept (11.527), the variance of the normally distributed random slopes

Output 12.16. Results of a logistic random coefficient analysis with both a random intercept and a random slope with time performed with MLwiN

$$\left. \begin{array}{l} \text{yvar01}_{ij} \sim \text{Binomial}(\text{denom}_{ij}, \pi_{ij}) \\ \text{yvar01}_{ij} = \pi_{ij} + e_{6ij}\,\text{bcons}* \end{array} \right\}$$

$\text{logit}(\pi_{ij}) = \beta_{0j}\text{cons} + \beta_{1j}\text{time}_{ij} + 0,384(1,303) \times 1_j +$
$0,655(0,119) \times 2_{ij} + -0,182(0,328) \times 3_{ij} + 0,269(0,565) \times 4_j$

$\beta_{0j} = -4,662(3,182) + u_{0j}$
$\beta_{1j} = -0,070(0,078) + u_{1j}$

$$\begin{bmatrix} u_{0j} \\ u_{1j} \end{bmatrix} \sim N(0,\ \Omega_u) \ : \ \Omega_u = \begin{bmatrix} 11,527(2,819) \\ -0,969(0,414) & 0,089(0,072) \end{bmatrix}$$

$\text{bcons}* = \text{bcons}[\pi_{ij}(1 - \pi_{ij})/\text{denom}_{ij}]^{0.5}$

$$\begin{bmatrix} e_{6ij} \end{bmatrix} \sim (0,\ \Omega_e) \ : \ \Omega_e = [1,000(0,000)]$$

with time (0.089) and the covariance between the random intercept and the random slope with time (−0.969). Besides this it can be seen that the overall error variance is fixed at a value of one, which is typical for a logistic random coefficient analysis.

It should also be noted that as a result of the PQL estimation procedure, no log likelihood values are produced. This is different from the Gauss–Hermite approach (implemented in SAS and STATA), which does produce a log likelihood value. So, with MLwiN the necessity of a random intercept or a random slope with time cannot be estimated with the likelihood ratio test. The only possibility left is to evaluate the magnitude of the different variances and the corresponding standard errors. Sometimes the standard deviation is divided by its standard error to obtain a sort of Wald statistic. However, although this provides some information about the necessity of a random coefficient, the interpretation is not straightforward. Logistic random coefficient analysis in MLwiN can be derived directly from the menu, so no syntax is needed.

12.5.5 Overview

Table 12.5 summarizes the results of the logistic random coefficient analysis with both a random intercept and a random slope with time performed with different software packages. From Table 12.5 it can be seen that there are major differences between the results obtained with the different software packages. Although the overall conclusions (if based on *p*-values) are the

Table 12.5. Summary of the results (i.e. regression coefficients, standard errors (in parentheses), and random variances) of a logistic random coefficient analysis with both a random intercept and a random slope with time performed with different software packages

	STATA[a]	SAS[b]	MLwiN[c]
X_1	0.33 (1.63)	0.15 (1.43)	0.38 (1.30)
X_2	0.72 (0.14)	0.72 (0.13)	0.66 (0.12)
X_3	−0.23 (0.36)	−0.19 (0.35)	−0.18 (0.33)
X_4	0.46 (0.70)	0.33 (0.63)	0.27 (0.57)
Time	−0.07 (0.10)	−0.04 (0.10)	−0.07 (0.08)
Random variance			
Intercept	13.116	15.905	11.527
Slope	0.109	0.138	0.089

[a] 12 quadrature points are used for the estimation.
[b] Nine quadrature points are used for the estimation.
[c] A second-order PQL procedure was used for the estimation.

same for all three analyses, the magnitude of the regression coefficients and standard errors is very different. It should also be noted that when a logistic random coefficient analysis is performed with the GLLAMM procedure in STATA with nine quadrature points, both the regression coefficients and the standard errors are different to those obtained with the NLMIXED procedure in SAS with nine quadrature points (results not shown in detail).

In general, a comparison between all logistic random coefficient analyses illustrated in this section indicates the instability of this kind of longitudinal analysis. In other words, the results obtained from a random coefficient analysis with dichotomous outcome variables must be interpreted very cautiously.

12.6 Categorical and 'count' outcome variables

Longitudinal data analysis with a categorical outcome variable is not implemented in many software packages yet. In the example discussed in Chapter 7, the GLLAMM procedure was used to analyse the longitudinal relationship between the categorical outcome variable Y_{cat} and the four predictor variables X_1 to X_4 and time. The syntax needed to perform that analysis is comparable to the syntax needed to perform other random coefficient analyses in STATA:

```
gllamm ycat x1 x2 x3 x4 time, i(id) fam(bin) link(mlogit)
nrf(2) eqs(int slope) nip(12)
```

The only difference from the syntax needed to perform a logistic random coefficient analysis is the fact that an mlogit link function is specified, which indicates that a multinominal (polytomous) logistic regression is performed.

All packages suitable for performing a logistic GEE analysis or a logistic random coefficient analysis are also suitable for the longitudinal analysis of a 'count' outcome variable. The only difference is that for the analysis of a 'count' outcome variable, a 'log' link function and a 'Poisson' distribution have to be specified. Although the output and syntax of the different packages will not be discussed in detail, just as an example the syntax needed for GEE analysis and random coefficient analysis with a 'count' outcome variable in STATA is given below:

```
xtgee ycount x1 x2 x3 x4 time, i(id) fam(poisson)
link(log) corr(exch)
gllamm ycount x1 x2 x3 x4 time, i(id) fam(poisson)
link(log) nrf(2) eqs(int slope) nip(12)
```

12.7 Alternative approach using covariance structures

Up to now, two sophisticated statistical techniques, developed to correct for the dependency of observations within one subject over time, have been discussed. There is, however, a widely used alternative approach for analysis of continuous outcome variables, which does not correct for within-subject **correlations**, but for within-subject **covariances** (see for instance Jennrich and Schluchter, 1986; Littel et al., 2000). In Section 4.7.3 it has already been mentioned that the covariance between an outcome variable measured twice in time is directly related to the correlation between the two measurements (Equation (4.10)).

The general concept of this approach is to select a priori a certain 'working' covariance structure, which is used in the estimation of the regression coefficients. It is not surprising that the possible choice of structures is comparable to the choice of correlation structures in GEE analysis (see Section 4.5.2). As in GEE analysis, one possibility is the 'independent structure', which models the covariances (i.e. correlations) as zero. The 'compound symmetry' or 'exchangeable covariance structure' assumes equal correlations (irrespective of the time interval between the repeated measurements), and equal variances of the repeated measurements. An 'exchangeable' covariance structure for a longitudinal study with six measurements is shown below:

$$\sigma^2 \times \begin{bmatrix} 1 & \rho & \rho & \rho & \rho & \rho \\ \rho & 1 & \rho & \rho & \rho & \rho \\ \rho & \rho & 1 & \rho & \rho & \rho \\ \rho & \rho & \rho & 1 & \rho & \rho \\ \rho & \rho & \rho & \rho & 1 & \rho \\ \rho & \rho & \rho & \rho & \rho & 1 \end{bmatrix}$$

Comparable to what has already been discussed for GEE analysis, several other structures can be chosen. For instance a 'first-order autoregressive covariance structure'

$$\sigma^2 \times \begin{bmatrix} 1 & \rho & \rho^2 & \rho^3 & \rho^4 & \rho^5 \\ \rho & 1 & \rho & \rho^2 & \rho^3 & \rho^4 \\ \rho^2 & \rho & 1 & \rho & \rho^2 & \rho^3 \\ \rho^3 & \rho^2 & \rho & 1 & \rho & \rho^2 \\ \rho^4 & \rho^3 & \rho^2 & \rho & 1 & \rho \\ \rho^5 & \rho^4 & \rho^3 & \rho^2 & \rho & 1 \end{bmatrix}$$

a '5-dependent covariance structure', which is also known as a 'Toeplitz (5) covariance structure'

$$\sigma^2 \times \begin{bmatrix} 1 & \rho_1 & \rho_2 & \rho_3 & \rho_4 & \rho_5 \\ \rho_1 & 1 & \rho_1 & \rho_2 & \rho_3 & \rho_4 \\ \rho_2 & \rho_1 & 1 & \rho_1 & \rho_2 & \rho_3 \\ \rho_3 & \rho_2 & \rho_1 & 1 & \rho_1 & \rho_2 \\ \rho_4 & \rho_3 & \rho_2 & \rho_1 & 1 & \rho_1 \\ \rho_5 & \rho_4 & \rho_3 & \rho_2 & \rho_1 & 1 \end{bmatrix}$$

an 'unstructured covariance structure'

$$\begin{bmatrix} \sigma_1{}^2 & \rho_{12}\sigma_1\sigma_2 & \rho_{13}\sigma_1\sigma_3 & \rho_{14}\sigma_1\sigma_4 & \rho_{15}\sigma_1\sigma_5 & \rho_{16}\sigma_1\sigma_6 \\ \rho_{12}\sigma_1\sigma_2 & \sigma_2{}^2 & \rho_{23}\sigma_2\sigma_3 & \rho_{24}\sigma_2\sigma_4 & \rho_{25}\sigma_2\sigma_5 & \rho_{26}\sigma_2\sigma_6 \\ \rho_{13}\sigma_1\sigma_3 & \rho_{23}\sigma_2\sigma_3 & \sigma_3{}^2 & \rho_{34}\sigma_3\sigma_4 & \rho_{35}\sigma_3\sigma_5 & \rho_{36}\sigma_3\sigma_6 \\ \rho_{14}\sigma_1\sigma_4 & \rho_{22}\sigma_2\sigma_4 & \rho_{34}\sigma_3\sigma_4 & \sigma_4{}^2 & \rho_{45}\sigma_4\sigma_5 & \rho_{46}\sigma_4\sigma_6 \\ \rho_{15}\sigma_1\sigma_5 & \rho_{25}\sigma_2\sigma_5 & \rho_{35}\sigma_3\sigma_5 & \rho_{45}\sigma_4\sigma_5 & \sigma_5{}^2 & \rho_{56}\sigma_5\sigma_6 \\ \rho_{16}\sigma_1\sigma_6 & \rho_{26}\sigma_2\sigma_6 & \rho_{36}\sigma_3\sigma_6 & \rho_{46}\sigma_4\sigma_6 & \rho_{56}\sigma_5\sigma_6 & \sigma_6{}^2 \end{bmatrix}$$

Although the unstructured covariance structure is obviously the best choice for the 'working' covariance structure, it can be seen that, when using this structure in a study with six measurements, 21 parameters must be calculated (six variance parameters and 15 correlation coefficients). As in GEE analysis, it is worthwhile to choose the least complicated covariance structure, which 'fits' the data well. It has already been mentioned that for GEE analysis there was no indication of the fit of the longitudinal model which could be used to evaluate the different correlation structures. In the approach based on covariance structures, however, the regression coefficients are estimated with maximum likelihood or restricted maximum likelihood, so models with different covariance structures can be compared by means of the log likelihoods.

12.7.1 Example

The alternative approach, correcting for the within-subject covariances, is implemented in the MIXED procedure in SAS, which was already discussed in Section 12.4.2, and in SPSS version 11 which was discussed in Section 12.4.4. Output 12.17 shows (a section of) the output of a longitudinal analysis with an unstructured covariance structure performed with the MIXED procedure in SAS.

The output looks similar to the output of the linear random coefficient analysis performed with the MIXED procedure in SAS. From the output it can be seen that 21 covariance parameters are estimated. The first parameter (UN(1,1)) is an indication of the variance of the first measurement, the second parameter (UN(2,1)) is an indication of the covariance between the first and the second measurements, and so on. It can also be seen that a restricted maximum likelihood (REML) estimation procedure is used, and that as a result of that a -2 res log likelihood is estimated (i.e. 1369.4). This value can

Output 12.17. Results of a longitudinal analysis with an unstructured covariance structure performed with the MIXED procedure in SAS

```
                    Model Information

Data Set                        LONGBOOK._FIRST_
Dependent Variable              YCONT
Covariance Structure            Unstructured
Subject Effect                  ID
Estimation Method               REML
Residual Variance Method        None
Fixed Effects SE Method         Model-Based
Degrees of Freedom Method       Between-Within

                       Dimensions
             Covariance Parameters          21
             Columns in X                    6
             Columns in Z                    0
             Subjects                      147
             Max Obs Per Subject             6
             Observations Used             882
             Observations Not Used           0
             Total Observations            882

            Covariance Parameter Estimates
            Cov Parm     Subject     Estimate
            UN(1,1)      ID          0.5044
            UN(2,1)      ID          0.3415
            UN(2,2)      ID          0.4187
            UN(3,1)      ID          0.2950
            UN(3,2)      ID          0.3242
            UN(3,3)      ID          0.4503
            UN(4,1)      ID          0.2356
            UN(4,2)      ID          0.3120
            UN(4,3)      ID          0.3799
            UN(4,4)      ID          0.4906
            UN(5,1)      ID          0.3222
            UN(5,2)      ID          0.2973
            UN(5,3)      ID          0.3113
            UN(5,4)      ID          0.2924
            UN(5,5)      ID          0.5305
            UN(6,1)      ID          0.4517
            UN(6,2)      ID          0.3490
            UN(6,3)      ID          0.3203
```

```
              UN(6,4)      ID           0.2208
              UN(6,5)      ID           0.4912
              UN(6,6)      ID           1.0840

                       Fit Statistics
          Res Log Likelihood                    -684.7
          Akaike's Information Criterion        -705.7
          Schwarz's Bayesian Criterion          -737.1
          -2 Res Log Likelihood                 1369.4

             Null Model Likelihood Ratio Test
               DF      Chi-Square     Pr > ChiSq
               20        625.87        <0.0001

                  Solution for Fixed Effects
                        Standard
   Effect      Estimate     Error    DF    t Value    Pr > |t|
   Intercept    3.8265      0.6616   144     5.78      <0.0001
   TIME         0.05719     0.01159  144     4.94      <0.0001
   X1          -0.05687     0.2716   144    -0.21       0.8344
   X2           0.1055      0.01946  144     5.42      <0.0001
   X3          -0.1041      0.05055  144    -2.06       0.0414
   X4           0.07004     0.1195   144     0.59       0.5587
```

be used to evaluate the necessity of an unstructured covariance structure in this particular situation. Again, it should be noted that the least complicated covariance structure is preferred. A possible next step is to analyse the same dataset with an exchangeable covariance structure. Output 12.18 shows the results of this analysis.

From the output it can be seen that with a compound symmetry (i.e. exchangeable) covariance structure only two covariance parameters are estimated. The likelihood ratio test can be used to decide which covariance structure is to be preferred in the analysis. Therefore, the difference between the -2 res log likelihoods of both models has to be calculated. This difference follows a χ^2 distribution with 19 degrees of freedom. Again, the number of degrees of freedom is based on the difference in the number of parameters to be calculated with each analysis. With the unstructured covariance structure, 21 parameters were calculated, while for the exchangeable covariance structure only two parameters were calculated. The difference between the -2 res log likelihoods (i.e. 220.7) is highly significant or, in other words, the

Output 12.18. Results of a longitudinal analysis with an exchangeable covariance structure performed with the MIXED procedure in SAS

```
Model Information
Data Set                          LONGBOOK._FIRST_
Dependent Variable                YCONT
Covariance Structure              Compound Symmetry
Subject Effect                    ID
Estimation Method                 REML
Residual Variance Method          Profile
Fixed Effects SE Method           Model-Based
Degrees of Freedom Method         Between-Within

            Covariance Parameters Estimates
            Cov Parm         Subject        Estimates
            CS               ID                0.3205
            Residual                           0.3205

                    Fit Statistics
        Res Log Likelihood                      -795.0
        Akaike's Information Criterion          -797.0
        Schwarz's Bayesian Criterion            -800.0
        -2 Res Log Likelihood                   1590.1

            Null Model Likelihood Ratio Test
            DF       Chi-Square       Pr > Chisq
            1          405.25          < 0.0001

            Solution for fixed Effects
                    Standard
Effect      Estimate      Error      DF    t Value    Pr > |t|
Intercept    3.6378      0.6786     144      5.36     <0.0001
TIME         0.1077      0.01106    732      9.74     <0.0001
X1          -0.03122     0.2784     144     -0.11      0.9109
X2           0.1102      0.02004    732      5.50     <0.0001
X3          -0.1140      0.05812    732     -1.96      0.0502
X4           0.09957     0.1226     144      0.81      0.4180
```

model with an unstructured covariance structure is 'better' than the model with an exchangeable covariance structure. Because there are other possible covariance structures that can be considered with less parameters to be estimated than with the unstructured covariance structure, the data were reanalysed with a 5-dependent (i.e. Toeplitz (5)) covariance structure, and

Table 12.6. −2 res log likelihoods and the number of estimated parameters of longitudinal data analysis correcting for different covariance structures

Covariance structure	−2 res log likelihood	Number of parameters estimated
Exchangeable (compound symmetry)	1590.1	2
First-order autoregressive	1541.2	2
5-Dependent (Toeplitz (5))	1504.4	6
Unstructured	1369.4	21

Table 12.7. Regression coefficients and standard errors (in parentheses) obtained from the SAS MIXED procedure correcting for different covariance structures and obtained from GEE analyses correcting for different correlation structures

	SAS MIXED (covariance structure)		GEE analysis (correlation structure)	
	Exchangeable	Unstructured	Exchangeable	Unstructured
X_1	−0.03 (0.28)	−0.06 (0.27)	−0.02 (0.27)	−0.01 (0.29)
X_2	0.11 (0.02)	0.11 (0.02)	0.11 (0.02)	0.11 (0.02)
X_3	−0.11 (0.06)	−0.10 (0.05)	−0.11 (0.06)	−0.09 (0.06)
X_4	0.10 (0.12)	0.07 (0.12)	0.10 (0.13)	0.09 (0.14)
Time	0.11 (0.01)	0.06 (0.01)	0.11 (0.01)	0.09 (0.01)

with a first-order autoregressive covariance structure. Table 12.6 summarizes the results.

Based on the results of the −2 res log likelihoods, an unstructured covariance structure seems to be the most appropriate in this particular situation. To illustrate the importance of a good choice of covariance structure, Table 12.7 shows the regression coefficients and standard errors of the four predictor variables and time, calculated with an exchangeable and an unstructured covariance structure. The same table also shows the coefficients for comparable GEE analyses.

From Table 12.7 it can be seen that the results of a GEE analysis with an exchangeable correlation structure are almost equal to the results obtained from an analysis using the MIXED procedure in SAS with an 'exchangeable' covariance structure. This is not surprising, because in both situations only one variance parameter and one correlation coefficient is estimated. The small difference observed in the results is due to the different estimation procedures (i.e. restricted maximum likelihood and quasi-likelihood). The major difference between the SAS MIXED procedure and the GEE analysis occurs in the comparison between an unstructured covariance and unstructured correlation structure. In the first situation, different variances are estimated at the different time-points, while in GEE analysis only one variance parameter is estimated. So (probably), the greatest advantage of the MIXED procedure, compared to GEE analysis, is the flexibility of modelling the variance over time. Furthermore, there is the possibility to evaluate the need for a certain (more complicated) covariance structure by means of the likelihood ratio test. A major disadvantage of the MIXED procedure in SAS is that it is only suitable for continuous outcome variables.

Finally, it should be noted that an analysis using the MIXED procedure in SAS with an 'exchangeable' covariance structure is exactly the same as a linear random coefficient analysis with only a random intercept. Comparing Output 12.18 with Output 12.7 in which the results of a linear random coefficient analysis with only a random intercept (estimated with restricted maximum likelihood) were provided, shows this.

The syntax needed to perform a longitudinal analysis with a correction for a unstructured covariance structure in the MIXED procedure is given below:

```
proc mixed data=long.x;
class id;
model ycont = x1 x2 x3 x4 time/s;
repeated id/ subject=id type=unstruc;
run;
```

The syntax is comparable to what has been discussed earlier for the MIXED procedure used to perform a linear random coefficient analysis. The differences are observed in the last line of the syntax, where the 'random' statement is replaced by the 'repeated' statement, and in the additional specification of the covariance structure (type=unstruc). A detailed description of the (almost infinite) possibilities within the SAS MIXED procedure can be found in the software manual (SAS Institute Inc., 1997).

Sample size calculations

13.1 Introduction

Before performing a (longitudinal) study, it is 'necessary' to calculate the number of subjects needed to ensure that a certain predefined effect is significant. Sample size calculations are also a prerequisite for research grants. This is basically a very strange phenomenon. First of all, sample size calculations are based on assumptions which can easily be changed, in which case the number of subjects needed will be totally different. Secondly, sample size calculations are related to the importance of 'significance levels' (how many subjects are needed to make a certain 'effect' **significant**?) and that is strange because in epidemiological research the importance of significance levels is becoming more and more questionable. Nevertheless there is a large amount of literature discussing sample size calculations in longitudinal studies (e.g. Lui and Cumberland, 1992; Snijders and Bosker, 1993; Lee and Durbin, 1994; Lipsitz and Fitzmaurice, 1994; Diggle et al., 1994; Liu and Liang, 1997; Hedeker et al., 1999).

However, because grant providers believe that sample size calculations are important, this chapter provides a few simple equations and some basic information on how to calculate sample sizes in longitudinal (experimental) studies.

Basically, the sample size calculations are the same as for 'standard' experimental studies. It should be noted that these 'standard' calculations are only suitable for experimental studies with one follow-up measurement. In fact, with the standard sample size calculations the difference in a certain outcome variable between several groups at the first follow-up measurement is used as an effect size. This assumes that the baseline values for the groups to be compared are equal, which is quite a reasonable assumption in a randomized trial. Equation (13.1) shows how the sample size can be calculated in the 'standard' situation for a continuous outcome variable.

$$N = \frac{\left(Z_{(1-\alpha/2)} + Z_{(1-\beta)}\right)^2 \sigma^2 (r+1)}{v^2 r} \tag{13.1}$$

where N is the sample size, $Z_{(1-\alpha/2)}$ is the $(1 - \alpha/2)$ percentile point of the standard normal distribution, $Z_{(1-\beta)}$ is the $(1 - \beta)$ percentile point of the standard normal distribution, σ is the standard deviation of the outcome variable, r is the ratio of the number of subjects in the compared groups, and v is the difference in mean value of the outcome variable between the groups.

For dichotomous outcome variables a comparable equation can be used (Equation (13.2)).

$$N = \frac{\left(Z_{(1-\alpha/2)} + Z_{(1-\beta)}\right)^2 \bar{p}(1 - \bar{p})(r+1)}{(p_1 - p_0)^2 r} \tag{13.2a}$$

$$\bar{p} = \frac{p_1 + (r p_0)}{1 + r} \tag{13.2b}$$

where N is the sample size, $Z_{(1-\alpha/2)}$ is the $(1 - \alpha/2)$ percentile point of the standard normal distribution, $Z_{(1-\beta)}$ is the $(1 - \beta)$ percentile point of the standard normal distribution, $\bar{p}$ is the 'weighted' average of p_0 and p_1, r is the ratio of the number of subjects in the compared groups, p_1 is the proportion of 'cases' in the intervention group, and p_0 is the proportion of 'cases' in the reference group.

When more than one follow-up measurement is carried out, and the purpose of the study is to compare the **development** in the outcome variable along the total follow-up period, the equations can be adjusted with an indication of the correlation between the repeated measurements (Equations (13.3) and (13.4)). It should be noted that when the purpose of the experimental study is just to compare the different groups at one single point in time, Equations (13.1) and (13.2) must be applied. For a continuous outcome variable the adjusted equation is as follows:

$$N = \frac{\left(Z_{(1-\alpha/2)} + Z_{(1-\beta)}\right)^2 \sigma^2 (r+1)[1 + (T-1)\rho]}{v^2 r T} \tag{13.3}$$

where N is the sample size, $Z_{(1-\alpha/2)}$ is the $(1 - \alpha/2)$ percentile point of the standard normal distribution, $Z_{(1-\beta)}$ is the $(1 - \beta)$ percentile point of the

Table 13.1. Sample sizes needed to make a certain difference in a continuous outcome variable statistically significant on a 5% level with a power of 80%; studies with different within-subject correlation coefficients (ρ)

	Expected difference (in standard deviation units)			
	0.1	0.2	0.5	1
Three repeated measurements				
$\rho = 0$	785	196	31	8
$\rho = 0.25$	981	245	39	10
$\rho = 0.5$	1178	294	47	12
Four repeated measurements				
$\rho = 0$	523	130	21	5
$\rho = 0.25$	785	196	31	8
$\rho = 0.5$	1047	262	42	10

standard normal distribution, σ is the standard deviation of the outcome variable, r is the ratio of the number of subjects in the compared groups, T is the number of **follow-up** measurements, ρ is the correlation coefficient of the repeated measurements, and v is the difference in mean value of the outcome variable between the groups.

To illustrate how many subjects are needed to show a certain significant difference between groups, Equation (13.3) is applied to several research situations in which the difference between groups is expressed in standard deviation units. Table 13.1 presents a 'sample size table' for several studies in which three and four measurements are carried out, i.e. in which two and three follow-up measurements are carried out.

For sample size calculations in experimental studies with a dichotomous outcome variable, Equation (13.4) can be applied:

$$N = \frac{\left(Z_{(1-\alpha/2)} + Z_{(1-\beta)}\right)^2 \bar{p}(1 - \bar{p})(r + 1)[1 + (T - 1)\rho]}{(p_1 - p_0)^2 r\, T} \tag{13.4}$$

where N is the sample size, $Z_{(1-\alpha/2)}$ is the $(1 - \alpha/2)$ percentile point of the standard normal distribution, $Z_{(1-\beta)}$ is the $(1 - \beta)$ percentile point of the standard normal distribution, $\bar{p}$ is the 'weighted' average of p_0 and p_1 (Equation (13.2b)), r is the ratio of the number of subjects in the compared

Table 13.2. Sample sizes needed to make a certain difference in a dichotomous outcome variable statistically significant on a 5% level with a power of 80%; studies with different within-subject correlation coefficients (ρ)

	Expected proportion of intervention group[a]		
	0.4	0.3	0.2
Three repeated measurements			
$\rho = 0$	194	47	20
$\rho = 0.25$	243	59	25
$\rho = 0.5$	291	71	30
Four repeated measurements			
$\rho = 0$	130	31	13
$\rho = 0.25$	194	47	20
$\rho = 0.5$	259	59	26

[a] The expected proportion in the reference category is assumed to be 0.5.

groups, T is the number of **follow-up** measurements, ρ is the correlation coefficient of the repeated measurements, p_1 is the proportion of 'cases' in the intervention group, and p_0 is the proportion of 'cases' in the reference group.

Based on Equation (13.4) a 'sample size table' for different studies with a dichotomous outcome variable can also be constructed (Table 13.2).

All sample size equations presented in this section can be used to estimate the sample size needed for a particular experimental study or to calculate the 'power' of that particular study. Here again it should be noted that for the calculation of sample sizes or power, certain assumptions are necessary, i.e. the expected difference between the groups, the standard deviation of the outcome variable of interest, and the within-subject correlation coefficient. Furthermore, in the equations, a specific significance level (usually 5%) is essential, and the importance of significance levels is rather doubtful. Caution is therefore strongly advised in the use of sample size equations.

13.2 Example

As has been mentioned before, Equations (13.3) and (13.4) can be used to calculate the power of a particular longitudinal study, given a certain sample size. In this section, power calculations will be performed for the two

Table 13.3. Information needed to perform a power analysis for an experimental study with a continuous outcome variable described in Section 9.2

N	average sample size at the first and second follow-up measurement, $N = 137$
sd	average standard deviation at the first and second follow-up measurement, sd $= 13.6$
ρ	correlation between the first and second follow-up measurement, $\rho = 0.687$
T	number of follow-up measurements, $T = 2$
$\left(Z_{(1-\alpha/2)} + Z_{(1-\beta)}\right)^2$	with a significance level of 5% and a power of 80%, $\left(Z_{(1-\alpha/2)} + Z_{(1-\beta)}\right)^2 = 7.85$

Table 13.4. Information needed to perform a power analysis for an experimental study with a dichotomous outcome variable described in Section 9.3

N	sample size per group, $N = 60$
p_0	proportion recovered in the reference group, $p_0 = 50\%$
ρ	correlation between the follow-up measurements (estimated with GEE analysis), $\rho = 0.15$
T	number of follow-up measurements, $T = 3$
$\left(Z_{(1-\alpha/2)} + Z_{(1-\beta)}\right)^2$	with a significance level of 5% and a power of 80%, $\left(Z_{(1-\alpha/2)} + Z_{(1-\beta)}\right)^2 = 7.85$

examples, which were explained in detail in Chapter 9. Table 13.3 shows the information that is needed to perform a power analysis for the experimental study with a continuous outcome variable.

With the information presented in Table 13.3, the smallest difference that will be significant in this experimental study can be calculated with Equation (13.3).

$$137 = \frac{7.85 \times 13.6^2 \times 2 \times [1 + (2 - 1) \times 0.687]}{v^2 \times 1 \times 2}$$

$$v = \sqrt{17.8789} = 4.23$$

So, the smallest difference in systolic blood pressure between the two groups that will be significant in this experimental study is 4.23 mmHg.

A similar calculation can be made for the example with a dichotomous outcome variable. Based on the information about the study (Table 13.4), the smallest detectable difference (i.e. the smallest difference to be significant) in proportions can be calculated:

$$60 = \frac{7.85 \times \bar{p}(1 - \bar{p}) \times 2 \times [1 + (3 - 1) \times 0.15]}{(p_1 - 0.50)^2 \times 1 \times 3}$$

$$\bar{p} = \frac{p_1 + (1 \times 0.50)}{1 + 1}$$

$$p_1 = \pm 0.335$$

In other words, with the characteristics of the experimental study with a dichotomous outcome variable presented in Chapter 9, a 16.5% (i.e. $50 - 33.5$) difference in proportion of recovery between the two groups will be significant at a 5% level.

References

Agresti, A., Booth, J.G., Hobart, J.P. and Caffo, B. (2000). Random-effects modelling of categorical response data. *Sociological Methodology*, **30**, 27–80.

Akaike, H. (1974). A new look at the statistical model identification. *IEEE Transactions on Automatic Control*, **19**, 716–23.

Albert, P.S. (1999). Longitudinal data analysis (repeated measures) in clinical trials. *Statistics in Medicine*, **18**, 1707–32.

Altman, D.G. (1991). *Practical statistics for medical research*. London: Chapman and Hall.

Barbosa, M.F. and Goldstein, H. (2000). Discrete response multilevel models for repeated measures: an application to intentions data. *Quality and Quantity*, **34**, 323–30.

Beunen, G., Lefevre, J., Claessens, A.L., Lysens, R., Maes, H., Renson, R., Simons, J., Vanden Eynde, B., Vanreusel, B. and Van Den Bossche, C. (1992). Age-specific correlation analysis of longitudinal physical fitness levels in men. *European Journal of Applied Physiology*, **64**, 538–45.

Blomquist, N. (1977). On the relation between change and initial value. *Journal of the American Statistical Association*, **72**, 746–9.

Bozdogan, H. (1987). Model selection and Akaike's information criterion (AIC): the general theory and its analytical extensions. *Psychometrika*, **52**, 345–70.

Breslow, N.E. and Clayton, D.G. (1993). Approximate inference in generalised linear models. *Journal of the American Statistical Association*, **88**, 9–25.

Burton, P., Gurrin, L. and Sly, P. (1998). Extending the simple linear regression model to account for correlated responses: an introduction to generalized estimating equations and multi-level mixed modelling. *Statistics in Medicine*, **17**, 1261–91.

Carey, V., Zeger, S.L. and Diggle, P.J. (1993). Modeling multivariate binary data with alternating logistic regression. *Biometrika*, **80**, 517–26.

Casey, V.A., Dwyer, J.T., Coleman, K.A. and Valadian, I. (1992). Body mass index from childhood to middle age: a 50-y follow-up. *American Journal of Clinical Nutrition*, **56**, 4–18.

Chen, P-L., Wong, E., Dominik, R. and Steiner, M.J. (2000). A transitional model of barrier methods compliance with unbalanced loss to follow-up. *Statistics in Medicine*, **19**, 71–82.

Clarke, W.R., Schrott, H.G., Leaverton, P.E., Connor, W.E. and Lauer, R.M. (1978). Tracking of blood lipids and blood pressures in school age children: the Muscatine Study. *Circulation*, **58**, 626–34.

Cohen, J. (1968). Weighted kappa: nominal scale agreement with provision for scaled disagreement or partial credit. *Psychological Bulletin*, **70**, 213–20.

Conway, M.R. (1990). A random effects model for binary data. *Biometrics*, **46**, 317–28.

Crowder, M.J. and Hand, D.J. (1990). *Analysis of repeated measures*. London: Chapman and Hall.

Deeg, D.J.H. and Westendorp-de Serière, M. (eds) (1994). *Autonomy and well-being in the aging population I: report from the Longitudinal Aging Study Amsterdam 1992–1993*. Amsterdam: VU University Press.

Diggle, P.J. (1989). Testing for random dropouts in repeated measurement data. *Biometrics*, **45**, 1255–8.

Diggle, P.J., Liang, K-Y. and Zeger, S.L. (1994). *Analysis of longitudinal data*. New York: Oxford University Press.

Dik, M.G., Jonker, C., Comijs, H.C., Bouter, L.M., Twisk, J.W.R., van Kamp, G.J. and Deeg, D.J.H. (2001). Memory complaints and Apo E ε4 accelerate cognitive decline in cognitively normal elderly. *Neurology*, **57**, 2217–22.

Fitzmaurice, G.M., Laird, N.M. and Lipsitz, S.R. (1994). Analysing incomplete longitudinal binary responses: a likelihood-based approach. *Biometrics*, **50**, 601–12.

Fleiss, J.L. (1981). *Statistical methods for rates and proportions*. New York: Wiley.

Foulkes, M.A. and Davis, C.E. (1981). An index of tracking for longitudinal data. *Biometrics*, **37**, 439–46.

Gebski, V., Leung, O., McNeil, D. and Lunn, D. (eds) (1992). *SPIDA user manual*, version 6. NSW, Australia: Macquarie University.

Gibbons, R.D. and Hedeker, D. (1997). Random effects probit and logistic regression models for three level data. *Biometrics*, **53**, 1527–37.

Goldstein, H. (1986). Multilevel mixed linear model analysis using iterative generalised least squares. *Biometrika*, **73**, 43–56.

Goldstein, H. (1989). Restricted unbiased iterative generalised least squares estimation. *Biometrika*, **76**, 622–3.

Goldstein, H. (1991). Nonlinear multilevel models with an application to discrete response data. *Biometrika*, **78**, 45–51.

Goldstein, H. (1995). *Multilevel statistical models*. London: Edward Arnold.

Goldstein, H. and Rasbash, J. (1996). Improved approximation for multilevel models with binary responses. *Journal of the Royal Statistical Society*, **159**, 505–13.

Goldstein, H., Rasbash, J., Plewis, I., Draper, D., Browne, W., Yang, M., Woodhouse, G. and Healy, M. (1998). *A user's guide to MLwiN*. London: Institute of Education.

Greenland, S. and Finkle, D. (1995). A critical look at methods for handling missing covariates in epidemiologic regression analysis. *American Journal of Epidemiology*, **142**, 1255–64.

Haan, M.N., Shemanski, L., Jagust, W.J., Manolio, T.A. and Kuller, L. (1999). The role of APOE ε4 in modulating effects of other risk factors for cognitive decline in elderly persons. *Journal of the American Medical Association*, **282**, 40–6.

Hand, D.J. and Crowder, M.J. (1996). *Practical longitudinal data analysis.* London: Chapman and Hall.

Harville, D.A. (1977). Maximum likelihood approaches to variance component estimation and to related problems. *Journal of the American Statistical Association,* **72**, 320–40.

Hedeker, D., Gibbons, R.D. and Waternaux, C. (1999). Sample size estimation for longitudinal designs with attrition: comparing time-related contrasts between groups. *Journal of Education and Behavioral Statistics,* **24**, 70–93.

Hibbert, M.E., Hudson, I.L., Lanigan, A., Landau, L.I. and Phelan, P.D. (1990). Tracking of lung function in healthy children and adolescents. *Pediatric Pulmonology,* **8**, 172–7.

van 't Hof, M.A. and Kowalski, C.J. (1979). Analysis of mixed longitudinal data-sets. In *A mixed longitudinal interdisciplinary study of growth and development,* ed. B. Prahl-Andersen, H.C.J. Kowalski and P. Heyendael, pp. 161–72. New York: Academic Press.

Hogan, J.W. and Laird, N.M. (1997). Mixture models for the joint distribution of repeated measures and event times. *Statistics in Medicine,* **16**, 239–57.

Holford, T.R. (1992). Analysing the temporal effects of age, period and cohort. *Statistical Methods in Medical Research,* **1**, 317–37.

Hosmer, D.W. and Lemeshow, S. (1989). *Applied logistic regression.* New York: Wiley.

Hu, F.B., Goldberg, J., Hedeker, D., Flay, B.R. and Pentz, M.A. (1998). Comparison of population-averaged and subject specific approaches for analyzing repeated measures binary outcomes. *American Journal of Epidemiology,* **147**, 694–703.

Hurvich, C.M. and Tsai, C-L. (1989). Regression and time series model selection in small samples. *Biometrika,* **76**, 297–307.

Jennrich, R.I. and Schluchter, M.D. (1986). Unbalanced repeated measures models with structured covariance matrices. *Biometrics,* **42**, 805–20.

Jöreskog, K.G. and Sörbom, D. (1993). *LISREL 8 user's reference guide.* Chicago, IL: Scientific Software International.

Jöreskog, K.G. and Sörbom, D. (2001). *LISREL 8.5.* Chicago, IL: Scientific Software International.

Judd, C.M., Smith, E.R. and Kidder, L.H. (1991). *Research methods in social relations.* Fort Worth, TX: Harcourt Brace Jovanovich College Publishers.

Kemper, H.C.G. (ed) (1995). *The Amsterdam growth study: a longitudinal analysis of health, fitness and lifestyle.* HK Sport Science Monograph Series, Vol. 6. Champaign IL: Human Kinetics Publishers.

Kenward, M.G. (1998). Selection models for repeated measurements with non-random dropout: an illustration of sensitivity. *Statistics in Medicine,* **17**, 2723–32.

Kenward, M.G. and Molenberghs, G. (1999). Parametric models for incomplete continuous and categorical longitudinal data. *Statistical Methods in Medical Research,* **8**, 51–84.

Kleinbaum, D.G. (1994). *Logistic regression. A self-learning text.* New York: Springer-Verlag.

Kwakkel, G., Wagenaar, R.C., Twisk, J.W.R., Lankhorst, G.J. and Koetsier, J.C. (1999). Intensity of leg and arm training after primary middle-cerebralartery stroke: a randomised trial. *Lancet,* **354**, 191–6.

Kupper, L.L., Janis, J.M., Karmous, A. and Greenberg, B.G. (1985). Statistical age–period–cohort analysis: a review and critique. *Journal of Chronic Diseases*, **38**, 811–30.

Laird, N.M. and Ware, J.H. (1982). Random effects models for longitudinal data. *Biometrics*, **38**, 963–74.

Lauer, R.M., Mahoney, L.T. and Clarke, W.R. (1986). Tracking of blood pressure during childhood: the Muscatine Study. *Clinical and Experimental Theory in Practice*, **A8**, 515–37.

Lebowitz, M.D. (1996). Age, period, and cohort effects. Influences on differences between cross-sectional and longitudinal pulmonary function results. *American Journal of Respiratory and Critical Care Medicine*, **154**, S273–7.

Lee, I-M., Paffenbarger Jr., R.S. and Hsieh, C-C. (1992). Time trends in physical activity among college alumni, 1962–1988. *American Journal of Epidemiology*, **135**, 915–25.

Lee, E.W. and Durbin, N. (1994). Estimation and sample size considerations for clustered binary responses. *Statistics in Medicine*, **13**, 1241–52.

Lesaffre, E. and Spiessens, B (2001). On the effect of the number of quadrature points in a logistic random-effects model: an example. *Applied Statistics*, **50**, 325–35.

Liang, K-Y. and Zeger, S.L. (1986). Longitudinal data analysis using generalised linear models. *Biometrica*, **73**, 45–51.

Liang, K-Y., Zeger, S.L. and Qaqish, B. (1992). Multivariate regression analysis for categorical data. *Journal of the Royal Statistical Society*, **54**, 3–40.

Liang, K-Y. and Zeger, S.L. (1993). Regression analysis for correlated data. *Annual Review of Public Health*, **14**, 43–68.

Lindsey, J.K. (1993). *Models for repeated measurements*. Oxford: Oxford University Press.

Lipsitz, S.R., Laird, N.M. and Harrington, D.P. (1991). Generalized estimating equations for correlated binary data: using the odds ratio as a measure of association. *Biometrika*, **78**, 153–60.

Lipsitz, S.R., Fitzmaurice, G.M., Orav, E.J. and Laird, N.M. (1994a). Performance of generalised estimating equations in practical situations. *Biometrics*, **50**, 270–8.

Lipsitz, S.R., Kim, K. and Zhao, L. (1994b). Analysis of repeated categorical data using generalised estimating equations. *Statistics in Medicine*, **13**, 1149–63.

Lipsitz, S.R. and Fitzmaurice, G.M. (1994). Sample size for repeated measures studies with binary repsonses. *Statistics in Medicine*, **13**, 1233–9.

Lipsitz, S.R. and Fitzmaurice, G.M. (1996). Estimating equations for measures of association between repeated binary responses. *Biometrics*, **52**, 903–12.

Littel, R.C., Freund, R.J. and Spector, P.C. (1991). *SAS system for linear models*, 3rd edn. Cary NC: SAS Institute Inc.

Littel, R.C., Milliken, G.A., Stroup, W.W. and Wolfinger, R.D. (1996). *SAS system for mixed models*. Cary, NC: SAS Institute Inc.

Littel, R.C., Pendergast, J. and Natarajan, R. (2000). Modelling covariance structures in the analysis of repeated measures data. *Statistics in Medicine*, **19**, 1793–1819.

Little, R.J.A. and Rubin, D.B. (1987). *Statistical analysis with missing data*. New York: Wiley.

Little, R.J.A. (1993). Pattern-mixture models for multivariate incomplete data. *Journal of the American Statistical Association*, **88**, 125–34.

Little, R.J.A. (1994). A class of pattern-mixture models for normal incomplete data. *Biometrika*, **81**, 471–83.

Little, R.J.A. (1995). Modelling the drop-out mechanism repeated measures studies. *Journal of the American Statistical Association*, **90**, 1112–21.

Liu, Q. and Pierce, D.A. (1994). A note on Gauss–Hermite quadrature. *Biometrika*, **81**, 624–9.

Liu, G. and Liang, K-Y. (1997). Sample size calculations for studies with correlated observations. *Biometrics*, **53**, 937–47.

Longford, N.T. (1993). *Random coefficient models*. Oxford: Oxford University Press.

Lui, K-J. and Cumberland, W.G. (1992). Sample size requirement for repeated measurements in continuous data. *Statistics in Medicine*, **11**, 633–41.

Mayer, K.U. and Huinink, J. (1990). Age, period, and cohort in the study of the life course: a comparison of classical A-P-C-analysis with event history analysis, or Farewell to Lexis? In *Data quality in longitudinal research*, ed. D. Magnusson and L.R. Bergman, pp. 211–32. Cambridge: Cambridge University Press.

MathSoft (2000). *S-PLUS 2000 guide to statistics*, Vol. 1. Data analysis product division. Seattle, WA: MathSoft Inc.

McCullagh, P. (1983). Quasi-likelihood functions. *Annals of Statistics*, **11**, 59–67.

McMahan, C.A. (1981). An index of tracking. *Biometrics*, **37**, 447–55.

McNally, R.J., Alexander, F.E., Strains, A. and Cartaright, R.A. (1997). A comparison of three methods of analysis age–period–cohort models with application to incidence data on non-Hodgkin's lymphoma. *International Journal of Epidemiology*, **26**, 32–46.

Miller, M.E., Davis, C.S. and Landis, J.R. (1993). The analysis of longitudinal polytomous data: generalized estimating equations and connections with weighted least squares. *Biometrics*, **49**, 1033–44.

Molenberghs, G., Michiels, B., Kenward, M.G. and Diggle, P.J. (1998). Monotone missing data and pattern-mixture models. *Statistica Neerlandica*, **52**, 153–61.

Nelder, J.A. and Pregibon, D. (1987). An extended quasi-likelihood function. *Biometrika*, **74**, 221–32.

Nelder, J.A. and Lee, Y. (1992). Likelihood, quasi-likelihood and psuedo-likelihood: some comparisons. *Journal of the Royal Statistical Society Series B*, **54**, 273–84.

Neuhaus, J.M., Kalbfleisch, J.D. and Hauck, W.W. (1991). A comparison of cluster-specific and population-averaged approaches for analyzing correlated binary data. *International Statistical Reviews*, **59**, 25–36.

NORM (1999). *Multiple imputation for incomplete multivariate data under a normal model. Software for Windows*. J.L. Schafer. University Park, PA: Department of Statistics, Pennsylvania State University.

Omar, R.Z., Wright, E.M., Turner, R.M. and Thompson, S.G. (1999). Thompson S.G. Analysing repeated measurements data: a practical comparison of methods. *Statistics in Medicine*, **18**, 1587–1603.

Pinheiro, J.C. and Bates, D.M. (1995). Approximations to the log-likelihood function in the non-linear mixed-effects model. *Journal of Computational and Graphical Statistics*, **4**, 12–35.

Pinheiro, J.C. and Bates, D.M. (2000). *Mixed-effects models in S and S-PLUS*. New York: Springer-Verlag.

Pockok, S.J. (1983). *Clinical trials: a practical approach*. Chichester: Wiley.

Porkka, K.V.K., Viikari, J.S.A. and Åkerblom, H.K. (1991). Tracking of serum HDL-cholesterol and other lipids in children and adolescents: the cardiovascular risk in young Finns study. *Preventive Medicine*, **20**, 713–24.

Prentice, R.L. (1988). Correlated binary regression with covariates specific to each binary observation. *Biometrics*, **44**, 1033–48.

Rabe-Hesketh, S. and Pickles, A. (1999). Generalised linear latent and mixed models. In *Proceedings of the 14th international workshop on statistical modelling*, ed. H. Friedl, A. Berghold and G. Kauermann, pp. 332–9. Graz, Austria.

Rabe-Hesketh, S., Pickles, A. and Taylor, C. (2000). sg129: generalized linear latent and mixed models. *Stata Technical Bulletin*, **53**, 47–57.

Rabe-Hesketh, S., Pickles, A. and Skrondal, A. (2001a). *GLAMM manual technical report 2001/01*. Department of Biostatistics and Computing, Institute of Psychiatry, King's College, University of London.

Rabe-Hesketh, S., Pickles, A. and Skrondal, A. (2001b). GLLAMM: a class of models and a Stata program. *Multilevel Modelling Newsletter*, **13** (1), 17–23.

Rabe-Hesketh, S. and Skrondal, A. (2001). Parameterisation of multivariate random effects models for categorical data. *Biometrics*, **57**, 1256–64.

Rasbash, J., Browne, W., Goldstein, H., Yang, M., Plewis, I., Healy, M., Woodhouse, G. and Draper, D. (1999). *A user's guide to MLwiN*, 2nd edn. London: Institute of Education.

Ridout, M.S. (1991). Testing for random dropouts in repeated measurement data. Reader reaction. *Biometrics*, **47**, 1617–21.

Robertson, C. and Boyle, P. (1998). Age–period–cohort analysis of chronic disease rates; I modelling approach. *Statistics in Medicine*, **17**, 1302–23.

Robertson, C., Gandini, S. and Boyle, P. (1999). Age–period–cohort models: a comparative study of available methodologies, *Journal of Clinical Epidemiology*, **52**, 569–83.

Rodriguez, G. and Goldman, N. (1995). An assessment of estimation procedures for multilevel models with binary responses. *Journal of the Royal Statistical Association*, **158**, 73–89.

Rodriguez, G. and Goldman, N. (2001). Improved estimation procedures for multilevel models with binary responses: a case study. *Journal of the Royal Statistical Association*, **164**, 339–55.

Rogossa, D. (1995). Myths and methods: "myths about longitudinal research" plus supplemental questions. In *The analysis of change*, ed. J.M. Gottman, pp. 3–66. Mahwah, NJ: Lawrence Erlbaum.

Rosner, B., Munoz, A., Tager, I., Speizer, F. and Weiss, S. (1985). The use of an autoregressive model for the analysis of longitudinal data in epidemiologic studies. *Statistics in Medicine*, **4**, 457–67.

Rosner, B. and Munoz, A. (1988). Autoregressive modelling for the analysis of longitudinal data with unequally spaced examinations. *Statistics in Medicine*, **7**, 59–71.

Rothman, K.J. and Greenland, S. (1998). *Modern epidemiology*. Philadelphia, PA: Lippincott-Raven.

Rubin, D.B. (1987). *Multiple imputation for nonresponse in surveys*. New York: Wiley.

Rubin, D.B. (1996). Multiple imputation after 18+ years. *Journal of the American Statistical Association*, **91**, 473–89.

SAS Institute Inc. (1997). *SAS/STAT software: changes and enhancements through release 6.12*. Cary, NC: SAS Institute Inc.

SAS Institute Inc. (2001). *SAS/STAT software: changes and enhancements, release 8.2*. Cary, NC: SAS Institute Inc.

Schafer, J.L. (1997). *Analysis of incomplete multivariate data*. New York: Chapman and Hall.

Schafer, J.L. (1999). Multiple imputation: a primer. *Statistical Methods in Medical Research*, **8**, 3–15.

Schall, R. (1991). Estimation in generalized linear models with random effects. *Biometrika*, **40**, 719–27.

Schwarz, G. (1978). Estimating the dimensions of a model. *Annals of Statistics*, **6**, 461–4.

Shih, W.J. and Quan, H. (1997). Testing for treatment differences with dropouts present in clinical trials – a composite approach. *Statistics in Medicine*, **16**, 1225–39.

Snijders, T.A.B. and Bosker, R.J. (1993). Standard errors and sample sizes for two-level research. *Journal of Educational Statistics*, **18**, 237–59.

SOLAS (1997). *SOLAS for missing data analysis*. Saugus, MA: Statistical Solutions, Stonehill Corporate Center.

SPSS (1997). *Statistical package for the social sciences, advanced statistics reference guide, release 7.5*. Chicago, IL: SPSS.

SPSS (1998). *Statistical package for the social sciences, SPSS 9.0 regression models*. Chicago, IL: SPSS.

Stanek III, E.J., Shetterley, S.S., Allen, L.H., Pelto, G.H. and Chavez, A. (1989). A cautionary note on the use of autoregressive models in analysis of longitudinal data. *Statistics in Medicine*, **8**, 1523–8.

STATA (2001). *Stata reference manual, release 7*. College Station, TX: Stata Press.

Stevens, J. (1996). *Applied multivariate statistics for the social sciences*, 3rd edn. Mahway, NJ: Lawrence Erlbaum.

Sun, J. and Song, P.X-K. (2001). Statistical analysis of repeated measurements with informative censoring times. *Statistics in Medicine*, **20**, 63–73.

Twisk, J.W.R., Kemper, H.C.G. and Mellenbergh, G.J. (1994). Mathematical and analytical aspects of tracking. *Epidemiological Reviews*, **16**, 165–83.

Twisk, J.W.R. (1997). Different statistical models to analyze epidemiological observational longitudinal data: an example from the Amsterdam Growth and Health Study. *International Journal of Sports Medicine*, **18** (Suppl. 3) S216–24.

Twisk, J.W.R., Kemper, H.C.G., van Mechelen, W. and Post, G.B. (1997). Tracking of risk factors for coronary heart disease over a 14 year period: a comparison between lifestyle and biological risk factors with data from the Amsterdam Growth and Health Study. *American Journal of Epidemiology*, **145**, 888–98.

Twisk, J.W.R., Staal, B.J., Brinkman, M.N., Kemper, H.C.G. and van Mechelen, W. (1998a). Tracking of lung function parameters and the longitudinal relationship with lifestyle. *European Respiratory Journal*, **12**, 627–34.

Twisk, J.W.R., Kemper, H.C.G., van Mechelen, W. and van Lenthe, F.J. (1998b). Longitudinal relationship of body mass index and the sum of skinfolds with other risk factors for coronary heart disease. *International Journal of Obesity*, **22**, 915–22.

Twisk, J.W.R., van Mechelen, W. and Kemper, H.C.G. (2000). Tracking of activity and fitness and the relationship with CVD risk factors. *Medicine Science in Sports and Exercise*, **32**, 1455–61.

Twisk, J.W.R., Kemper, H.C.G., van Mechelen, W. and Post, G.B. (2001). Clustering of risk factors for coronary heart disease. The longitudinal relationship with lifestyle. *Annals of Epidemiology*, **11**, 157–65.

Twisk, J.W.R. and de Vente, W. (2002). Attrition in longitudinal studies. How to deal with missing data. *Journal of Clinical Epidemiology*, **55**, 329–37.

Venables, W.N. and Ripley, B.D. (1997). *Modern applied statistics with S-PLUS*, 2nd edn. New York: Springer-Verlag.

Verbeke, G. and Molenberghs, G. (2000). *Linear mixed models for longitudinal data*. New York: Springer-Verlag.

Vermeulen, E.G.J., Stehouwer, C.D.A., Twisk, J.W.R., van den Berg, M., de Jong, S., Mackaay, A.J.C., van Campen, C.M.C., Visser, F.J., Jakobs, C.A.J.M., Bulterijs, E.J. and Rauwerda, J.A. (2000). Effect of homocysteine-lowering treatment with folic acid plus vitamin B6 on progression of subclinical atherosclerosis: a randomised, placebo-controlled trial. *Lancet*, **355**, 517–22.

Ware, J.H. and Wu, M.C. (1981). Tracking: prediction of future values from serial measurements. *Biometrics*, **37**, 427–37.

Wiliamson, J.M., Kim, K. and Lipsitz, S.R. (1995). Analyzing bivariate ordinal data using a global odds ratio. *Journal of the American Statistical Association*, **90**, 1432–7.

Wolfinger, R., Tobias, R. and Sall, J. (1994). Computing Gaussian likelihoods and their derivates for general linear mixed models. *SIAM Journal of Scientific Computation*, **15**, 1294–310.

Wolfinger, R.D. (1998). Towards practical application of generalized linear mixed models. In *Proceedings of the 13th international workshop on statistical modelling*, ed. B. Marx and H. Friedl, pp. 388–95. New Orleans, LA.

Yang, M. and Goldstein, H. (2000). Multilevel models for repeated binary outcomes: attitudes and voting over the electoral cycle. *Journal of the Royal Statistical Society*, **163**, 49–62.

Zeger, S.L. and Liang, K-Y. (1986). Longitudinal data analysis for discrete and continuous outcomes. *Biometrics*, **42**, 121–30.

Zeger, S.L. and Qaqish, B. (1988). Markov regression models for time series: a quasi-likelihood approach. *Biometrics*, **44**, 1019–31.

Zeger, S.L., Liang, K-Y. and Albert, P.S. (1988). Models for longitudinal data: a generalised estimating equation approach. *Biometrics*, **44**, 1049–60.

Zeger, S.L. and Liang, K-Y. (1992). An overview of methods for the analysis of longitudinal data. *Statistics in Medicine*, **11**, 1825–39.

Index